IMPROVE YOUR DIGESTION

Other books by Patrick Holford

The Optimum Nutrition Bible
The Optimum Nutrition Cookbook (with Judy Ridgway)
100% Health
Beat Stress and Fatigue
Boost Your Immune System (with Jennifer Meek)
Say No to Cancer
Say No to Heart Disease
Balancing Hormones Naturally (with Kate Neil)
The 30-Day Fatburner Diet
The Whole Health Manual
Mental Health and Illness – The Nutrition Connection

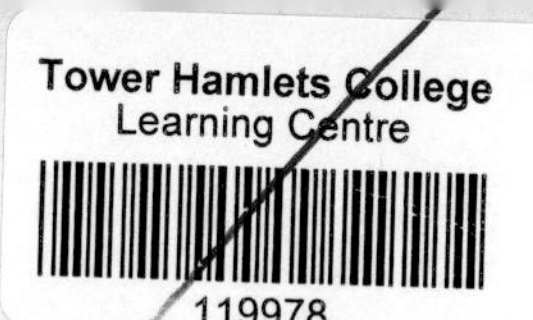

IMPROVE YOUR DIGESTION

PATRICK HOLFORD

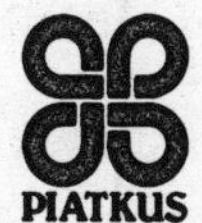

PIATKUS

First published in Great Britain in 1999 by Piatkus Books
This paperback edition published in 1999 by Piatkus Books

Reprinted eight times
Reprinted 2006, 2007, 2008

A CIP catalogue record for this book is available from the British Library

ISBN 978-0-7499-2014-2

Designed by Paul Saunders
Illustrations by Jonathan Phillips

Printed and bound in Great Britain by
Mackays of Chatham Ltd, Chatham, Kent

Piatkus Books
An imprint of
Little, Brown Book Group
100 Victoria Embankment
London EC4Y 0DY

An Hachette Livre UK Company

www.piatkus.co.uk

CONTENTS

PART 3 DIGESTIVE PROBLEMS AND SOLUTIONS

PART 4 RESTORING DIGESTIVE HEALTH

ACKNOWLEDGEMENTS

Many people have helped research, check and edit this book. Special thanks go to Brian Wright for his help and expertise regarding colon cleansing, to Antony Haynes for his help regarding digestive infections and to Erica White for her help on new approaches to candidiasis. Most of all, I am indebted to my sub-editor Natalie Savona, who also contributed the chapters on irritable bowel and leaky gut syndrome. Also thanks to the wonderful editorial team at Piatkus, Rachel Winning and Kelly Davis.

Guide to abbreviations and measures

1 gram (g) = 1000 milligrams (mg) = 1 000 000 micrograms (mcg or µg).
Most vitamins are measured in milligrams or micrograms. Vitamins A, D and E are also measured in International Units (iu), a measurement designed to standardise the different forms of these vitamins which have different potencies.
1mcg of retinol (mcgRE) = 3.3iu of vitamin A (RE = Retinol Equivalents)
1mcg RE of beta-carotene = 6mcg of beta-carotene
100iu of vitamin D = 2.5mcg
100iu of vitamin E = 67mg
1 pound (lb) = 16 ounces (oz)   2.2lb = 1 kilogram (kg)
In this book calories means kilocalories (kcals)

References and further sources of information

Hundreds of references from respected scientific literature have been used in writing this book. Details of specific studies referred to are listed on pages 170–173. Other supporting research for statements made is available from the Lamberts Library at the Institute for Optimum Nutrition (ION) (see page 176). Members are free to visit and study there. ION also offers information services, including literature search and library search facilities, for those readers who want to access the scientific literature on specific subjects. On page 174 you will also find Recommended Reading which suggests the best books to read if you wish to dig deeper into the topics covered.

INTRODUCTION

Contrary to popular belief, you are not what you eat. You are what you can digest and absorb. Nothing is more important to your overall health than the health of your digestive tract. It is the interface between your body and the outside world. Over a lifetime, no less than 100 tons of food pass along the digestive tract. The digestive tract is your 'inside skin' and represents a 10-metre-long tube with a surface area the size of a small football pitch. Amazingly, most of the billions of cells that make up this barrier between your body and the environment are renewed every four days.

We, like other animals, spend our physical lives processing organic matter, extracting nutrients, building materials and fuel, and eliminating the rest. How good we are at this determines our energy level, longevity and state of body and mind. A professor at the Harvard School of Medicine once rightly said, 'A strong stomach and a good set of bowels are more important to human happiness than a large amount of brains.'

The digestive tract is the gateway into the body, jealously guarded by an immune army, kept healthy by a careful balance of millions of benign bacteria. Before food is ready to be presented to the inner kingdom of the body, it must be prepared, broken down, digested. Only then can it be invited to enter as a welcome guest.

Before birth children are connected to their mothers and receive nourishment directly into their bloodstream. At birth the umbilical cord is cut and the digestive system takes over, but the infants are still reliant on their mothers to provide nourishment. As we take over our own nourishment we lose that maternal dependence but we are still totally dependent on our food. Our very survival depends on it. No wonder so many religions advocate starting each meal with a prayer – an act of remembering the relationship between food, us and the source of provision.

Our senses of sight, touch taste and smell help guide us towards that which is nourishing in the natural world. Nowadays, however, our senses, cleverly manipulated by artificially coloured, flavour-enhanced and sweetened convenience foods, have become our masters.

We have, for example, a need for essential fats. In our mouths, accordingly, are fat receptors that respond to the ingestion of essential fats. If, on the other hand, we eat saturated fat or fake fats designed to simulate the texture of fat, the fat receptors are not so strongly stimulated and do not pass on the message of satisfaction. Consequently, we continue to crave fat and continue to choose the wrong kind of fat, causing ourselves many long-term health problems.

Taking in all the nutrients we need at optimal amounts is not only a recipe for a long and healthy physical life, but also helps us achieve our full potential as human beings. Because the body knows when it is receiving everything it requires for its survival, our energy and consciousness can be directed towards fulfilling other needs.

The consequences of sub-optimum nutrition are evident in the increasing incidence of digestive problems and diseases. There is no doubt that many of us are digging our own graves with a knife and fork. No longer is most of society's suffering as a result of poverty. Indeed, much of the Western world's illness is the consequence of eating too much, rather than too little, and eating the wrong kinds of food.

As a result, there is a quiet epidemic of digestive problems, including indigestion, irritable bowel syndrome, stomach bugs, ulcers, Crohn's, colitis and diverticulitis, candidiasis and chronic fatigue.

Whether or not you are currently suffering from any of these ailments, the chances are that you could tune up your digestion and reap rewards in terms of extra health and energy. This book is designed to help you do just that. Parts 1 and 2 explain the digestive system, from the beginnings of digesting your food to the act of absorbing nutrients into the body, describing each step along the way, what goes wrong and how you can adjust your eating to ensure optimal digestion and absorption.

Part 3 focuses on specific digestive problems and solutions that can help restore your digestive health. Part 4 puts it all together into an action plan that you can use to clean up your act, detoxify your body and experience the consistent energy and clarity of mind that come from optimally nourishing yourself.

PART 1

IMPROVING DIGESTION

CHAPTER 1

THE DIGESTIVE SYSTEM – A GUIDED TOUR

The human body is essentially a ring doughnut. In the digestive tract (the hole in the middle) large food particles are broken down into smaller ones, which can then be absorbed into the body. The digestive tract (technically known as the gastro-intestinal tract) is around 10 metres long and has various organs attached to it which produce digestive juices.

THE STAGES OF DIGESTION

The mouth

Digestion starts in the mouth where the act of chewing food starts to physically break it down. Leading into the mouth are salivary glands which produce saliva. Saliva has a dual role: lubricating the food to make it easy to swallow and also starting the process of digestion. Saliva is rich in a digestive enzyme called ptyalin which can break down carbohydrate. Food then passes down the throat, along the oesophagus and into the stomach.

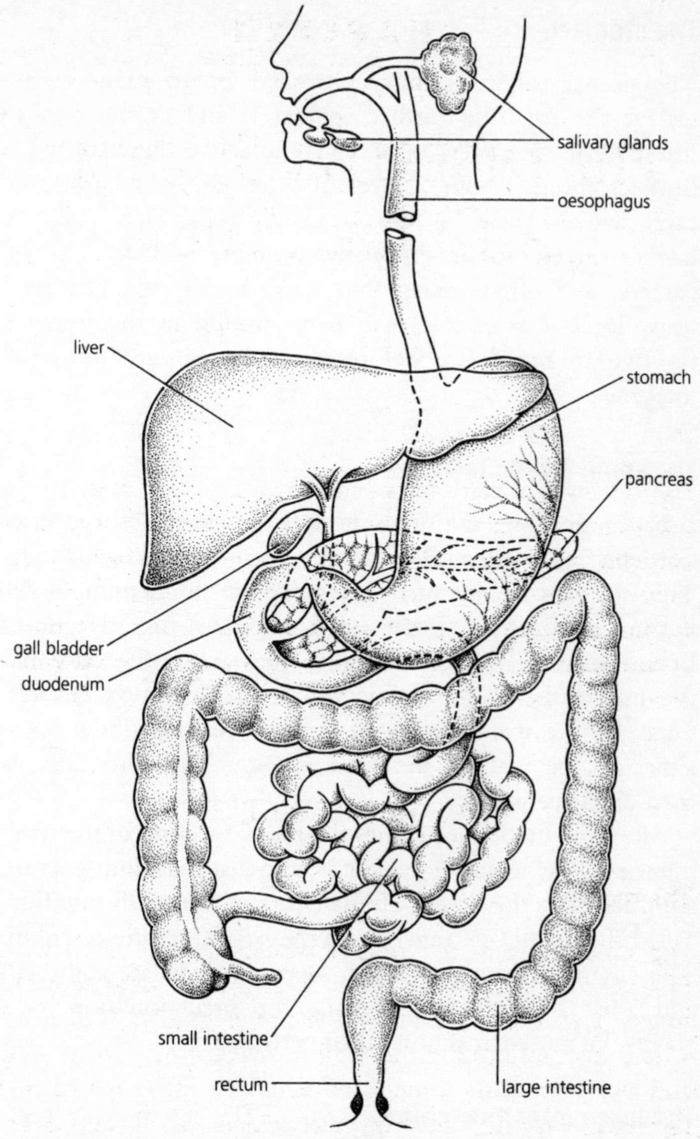

Figure 1 – The digestive system

The stomach

The stomach is a carefully controlled environment with a seal at the top (the cardiac sphincter) and at the bottom (the pyloric sphincter) to prevent the acidic digestive juices from escaping. About 2 litres of these juices are produced each day by cells in the stomach wall. They help to further digest food, especially protein, and to kill off bacteria and other undesirable micro-organisms. The food (now known as chyme) can hang around in the stomach for two to five hours before it is released into the small intestine.

The small intestine

Broadly speaking, the small intestine is where absorption of nutrients takes place. But this doesn't happen immediately. The first part of the small intestine, the duodenum, is the hotspot of digestion, because it is here that digestive juices from the liver and pancreas pour in via the bile duct and the pancreatic duct. As you will see in the next chapter, these are the main players in further breaking down food, although the wall of the small intestine also produces its own digestive juices.

After the duodenum comes the middle section of the small intestine – the jejunum – and it is here that most nutrients are absorbed into the body. The last part of the small intestine, called the ileum, is connected to the large intestine or colon. The chyme is further digested, more nutrients are absorbed, and what is left is passed along the small intestine by a wave-like muscular action called peristalsis.

The large intestine (colon)

While the small intestine is primarily involved in digestion and absorption, the large intestine prepares what is left (mainly undigested fibres, unabsorbed food, bacteria and dead cells) for elimination. These two areas – the 'kitchen' area and the 'waste' area – are kept separate by a muscular seal called the ileo-caecal valve. If this valve doesn't work properly there is a danger that undesirable organisms will move from the large into the small intestine, leading to intestinal infections (see pages 87–93).

Although some nutrients are absorbed from the colon, its main role is to re-absorb water from the chyme and pass waste material along, ready for elimination. About a litre of water a day is re-absorbed in this way. Again, peristaltic muscle contractions help to move material along into the rectum, the last part of the colon. When this is full, it triggers defecation.

As well as eliminating unabsorbed food matter, defecation also gets rid of other substances from the body, including dead blood cells and cholesterol.

TACKLING DIGESTIVE PROBLEMS

Digestive problems are best considered by asking three fundamental questions: Are you digesting your food properly? Are you absorbing properly? Are you eliminating properly? These three stages – digestion, absorption and elimination – don't just apply to physical material. After all, isn't this what we do with psychological material too? When you read a newspaper, for example, you digest certain stories, absorb some facts or ideas, then eliminate the rest. Quite often people who have physical problems with elimination also find it difficult to let go of things, both physically and mentally. They may hoard unnecessary psychological baggage.

When tuning up your digestion it's best to work from the top down. For this reason the next chapter looks at the first key process, chewing, followed by digestion and the role of digestive enzymes.

In each chapter there are simple guidelines for you to follow to improve your digestion. With current testing methods and recent advances in natural treatments, the vast majority of digestive problems can be solved with relative ease, little expense and no need for invasive tests or treatment. A survey of patients who had seen a clinical nutritionist reported a greater than 90 per cent success rate in relieving digestive problems.[1] The digestive tract is one of the most regenerative parts of the body and, with the right diet, the majority of digestive problems can be swiftly resolved. For those without any apparent digestive problems, following the guidelines in this book may further improve your ability to derive energy from food, thus increasing your vitality and resistance to disease.

CHAPTER 2

IT'S GOOD TO CHEW

As simple as it may sound, the act of digesting and absorbing nutrients from food is a highly complex and carefully orchestrated affair. As soon as you think about food, see it, smell it and taste it, the digestive tract starts preparing the right digestive juices to deal with the meal. Given that the body produces 10 litres of digestive juices every day, how does it know what to produce? If you eat protein rather than carbohydrate, or a large meal rather than a small meal, the amount and type of digestive juices needed will be very different. And how does the body know if a food is good or bad for you? These questions are being answered even before you swallow a piece of food.

First, your eyes recognise what is edible and attractive. Much more powerful is the nose. Smell literally involves taking in tiny particles of the food. If a food has gone bad it may not always look bad, but it will certainly smell bad. That's why no animal ever eats a piece of food without smelling it first. As food enters your mouth the nature of the food is being analysed, which triggers the production and release of different digestive enzymes. This process is helped by smelling and chewing your food. Sometimes people get indigestion just because they wolf their food down without chewing it.

Chewing does much more than just signal what's to come. The salivary glands in the mouth release large amounts of saliva which contains the digestive enzyme ptyalin. Ptyalin helps to break down large carbohydrate particles into smaller ones (which is why, if you keep chewing a piece of bread, it will actually get digested in your mouth). So, the more you chew, the better you prepare food by pre-digesting it, and the less work your digestive system has to do. Obviously, chewing also physically breaks down food into smaller pieces, increasing the surface area of your food and making it easier for the digestive juices to do their work.

GUT REACTIONS

The digestive system does much more than digest food. Scientists are discovering that the digestive system 'thinks' and 'feels' and may act almost as a second brain. Early models of the brain and cognition proposed that what we call thinking and feeling boiled down to the sending and receiving of chemical messengers called neuro-transmitters and hormones. Now scientists are discovering that there is a vast amount of neuro-transmitter and hormone activity in the digestive tract. In addition to this, there are more immune cells in the gut than there are in the rest of the body. These three – neuro-transmitters, hormones and immune cells – are the chemicals of communication of what is now known as the neuro-endo-immune system, or, to put it simply, the intelligence of the body. It is this highly sophisticated network that allows us to keep responding appropriately to our ever-changing environment.

In practical terms, this means that you can't separate thoughts, feelings and physical reactions. What you eat, what you think and feel about *what* you eat, and what you think and feel about *when* you eat, all have a bearing on the end result. This is why, for optimum nourishment, it is good to choose the best foods, prepare them in a way that you like, eat the food consciously, and have good thoughts as you are actually eating.

This is the complete opposite of modern eating which usually takes place in the fast lane. Often, when I ask clients what they have eaten in the last two days they struggle to remember. Lunch was something grabbed from a sandwich shop and eaten unconsciously, amid stressful thoughts and feelings. Much of today's food is eaten on the run. How different this is from the culture of Mediterranean countries where everyone helps to prepare the food, and to set the table, while family and friends take time to enjoy the feast. No wonder they have fewer heart attacks!

So, next time you eat a meal:

- Select high-quality foods and prepare them so that they look and taste good.
- Smell your food before you eat it.
- Think about its origin and that these molecules of food will literally become you.
- Remember to chew each mouthful completely before beginning the next.
- Take some time off for your meals and either eat alone or in good company.

CHAPTER 3

ENZYMES – THE KEYS OF LIFE

The food we eat is made out of large, complex molecules that can't possibly enter out bodies. First they have to be broken down into much smaller particles which are not only physically able to get through the wall of the digestive tract but are also 'on the guest list'. This breaking down process is the job of digestive enzymes.

These enzymes are produced in large amounts at different stages along the digestive tract. If you don't produce enough of them to digest your food, you can get indigestion, bloating and flatulence. The long-term effects of having undigested food in your system, however, are more insidious and can lead to a greater risk of inflammatory bowel syndrome, digestive infections (such as candidiasis) and allergies.

DIGESTING CARBOHYDRATE

Carbohydrate digestion begins in the mouth, through the action of the enzyme ptyalin. Ptyalin is an amylase (an enzyme that digests carbohydrate). Carbohydrate doesn't get further digested in the stomach, so it can theoretically pass straight into the duodenum (the first part of the small

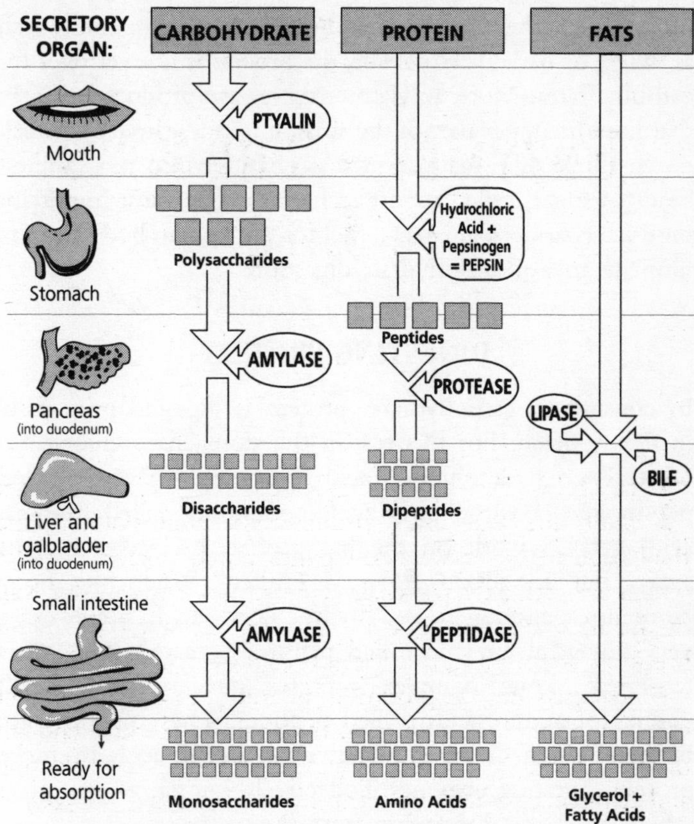

Figure 2 – Digestive enzymes

intestine), which is where the fun starts as far as carbohydrates are concerned.

Special cells in the pancreas produce large amounts of amylase enzymes that pour out of the pancreatic duct into the duodenum, ready to break down carbohydrate. The pancreas also produces alkaline substances that help to neutralise the acid that was mixed into the food in the stomach. Amylase enzymes break down complex sugar molecules called polysaccharides (for example in grains) into simpler sugars such as malt (the sugar that can be produced from grains such as wheat or barley). However, the process is not yet over for carbohydrates. More amylase enzymes are produced in cells that line the upper part of the small intestine; these can break down things like maltose (a disaccharide) into the simplest kinds of sugar, called monosaccharides. The most important monosaccharide is glucose – fuel for the human body and the ultimate goal of carbohydrate digestion.

DIGESTING PROTEIN

In contrast to carbohydrate, protein is digested principally in the stomach. For this reason the stomach produces two substances: hydrochloric acid and an enzyme called pepsinogen. Hydrochloric acid (commonly called stomach acid) gets to work on the big protein molecules straight away, but its action alone is limited. When the body combines pepsinogen and hydrochloric acid, however, a very powerful enzyme called pepsin is created. This starts to break down complex proteins into relatively small chunks of amino acids, called peptides. These peptides are further broken down into individual amino acids by more protein-digesting enzymes (collectively known as proteases) which enter the duodenum from the pancreas.

Protein digestion is also done by protease enzymes produced by special cells in the first part of the small intestine. The end result, if all goes well, is that complex proteins end up as simple amino acids, ready for absorption.

DIGESTING FAT

Fat is a whole different ball game. While protein and carbohydrate are effectively water-soluble and can therefore be acted on by the enzymes in digestive juices, fat repels water and is thus impervious to these enzymes. For this reason, the first stage of digesting fat, called emulsification, is all about actually preparing fat particles for digestion. This is done by a substance called bile which is made in the liver and stored in the gall bladder. What bile does is break down large fat globules into tiny droplets of fat. The consequence of effectively turning a football into 15 tennis balls is that there is a much greater surface area exposed to digestive juices. Once again, the pancreas plays a key role because the digestive juices it produces and sends into the duodenum contain lipase, a fat-digesting enzyme.

So, on the one hand, bile enters the duodenum along the bile duct, and starts to break the fat into tiny particles. Meanwhile, lipase enters the duodenum which actually digests the fat, ready for absorption.

Bile (produced by the liver and concentrated in the gall bladder) is a combination of alkaline salts which help to neutralise stomach acid, lecithin (the primary emulsifying factor) and cholesterol. Whenever you eat fat, the body gets ready by squeezing the gall bladder to secrete bile into the digestive tract. If you've had your gall bladder removed, the liver still produces bile but it's not nearly as concentrated and isn't automatically released when you eat fat. This means that you can still digest some fat but not so much, so it is important to eat a consistently low-fat diet. One way to improve matters is to supplement lecithin with any meal containing fat, as lecithin is the main emulsifying agent which prepares fat for digestion. Lecithin is available either as granules (in which case you simply add a dessert spoonful to each meal) or as capsules (in which case you take 1200mg with each meal).

SOLVING INDIGESTION

One of the main reasons for indigestion is that the person doesn't produce enough of all these enzymes to digest their food properly. This means that incompletely digested food hangs around in the small intestine, feeding the bacteria that live there. These bacteria produce gas, resulting in bloating, flatulence and digestive pain. Stomach acid release can also be a problem (see Chapter 5). If a person has particular difficulty digesting fat, the stools tend to be very buoyant and light in colour. Also, since the goodness in the food isn't getting into the body, instead of feeling better after a meal such a person often feels worse.

The body cells, such as those in the pancreas, depend on vitamins and minerals to produce enzymes. But if you're not digesting your food you don't get the nutrients you need to make these enzymes – so it's a vicious circle. Nowadays it is relatively easy to find out if a person isn't digesting properly, using two non-invasive tests. The first, known as the Gastrogram, was invented by Dr John McLaren Howard at Biolab in London (see Useful Addresses). It involves swallowing special capsules which transmit messages showing the efficiency of stomach acid secretion, the speed at which the stomach is emptying into the small intestine, and the efficiency of pancreatic enzymes. The other method is stool analysis (see Useful Addresses for stool test laboratories). If the stool contains undigested protein, fats or carbohydrates this can also identify a digestion problem.

The first action to take if you've got indigestion is to supplement digestive enzymes, the main three being amylase, protease and lipase. Digestive enzymes come in many different forms, ranging from natural compounds (rich in one or other enzyme) to combinations of amylase, protease and lipase. Here are the common ingredients you might find in a digestive enzyme supplement:

Enzymes naturally present in raw foods

	Digests Fat	Digests Protein	Digests Carbohydrate
Papain (from papaya)		√	
Bromelain (from pineapple)	√	√	
Pancreatin (extract of pancreas)	√	√	√
Ox bile extract	√		
Amylase			√
Protease		√	
Lipase	√		

Some digestive enzymes also contain lactase, which is the enzyme for digesting lactose, the primary sugar in milk. Others contain an additional enzyme called alpha-galactosidase. This enzyme helps to digest some of the naturally indigestible compounds found in certain vegetables and beans, hence preventing wind. Another key ingredient is betaine hydrochloride, which is stomach acid. Whether or not you need a supplement containing this is discussed fully in the next chapter. Some supplements also contain amylo-glucosidase which helps to digest glucosides found in cruciferous vegetables such as cabbage, kale, cauliflower, broccoli and Brussels sprouts, thereby reducing wind.

If you're vegetarian it's best to choose a digestive enzyme supplement that provides amylase, protease and lipase. If you're not, pancreatin is a safe bet.

You can test the effects of these enzyme supplements by crushing them and stirring them into a thick porridge. If the product is good the porridge will become liquid in 30 minutes. While there is no harm in taking digestive enzymes on an ongoing basis, correcting digestive enzyme levels with supplements paves the way for increasing body levels of nutrients. Once this is achieved, digestion often improves of its own accord and then the digestive enzyme supplements may no longer be necessary. For this reason I'd recommend taking a digestive enzyme supplement with each main meal for a month, then stopping. If lack of enzymes is a problem you should start to feel relief in the first few days.

ENZYME-FRIENDLY FOODS

Problems with digestion aren't just about lack of digestive enzymes. If you over-eat this is going to strain your body's ability to digest even under the best of circumstances. Therefore grazing rather than gorging – eating little and often – is a great help to digestion. So too is eating raw foods. Raw foods contain significant amounts of enzymes. Professor Artturi Virtanen, Helsinki biochemist and Nobel prize winner, showed that enzymes in uncooked foods are released in the mouth when vegetables are chewed. When these foods are crushed, the enzymes come into contact with the food and start the act of digestion.

These food enzymes are not denatured by stomach acid, as some researchers have suggested, but in fact remain active throughout the digestive tract. Extensive tests by Kaspar Tropp in Wurzburg have shown that the human body has a way of protecting enzymes that pass through the gut so that more than half reach the colon intact. There they alter the intestinal flora by binding free oxygen, reducing the chances of fermentation and putrefaction in the intestines (a factor linked to cancer of the colon). In so doing they also help to create conditions in which lactic-acid-forming beneficial bacteria can grow.

Some foods also contain enzyme blockers. For example, lentils, beans and chickpeas contain trypsin-inhibitors (preventing protein from complete digestion), which is why they can produce a lot of gas. However, this anti-enzyme factor is destroyed either by sprouting the food or by cooking it.

The two main digestive enzymes, amylase and protease, are found in many foods. For centuries, man has put these food enzymes to work by pre-digesting foods before eating them. Fermented foods, such as yoghurt or sauerkraut, are examples of this. However, raw foods also contain these enzymes, which become active when we chew but are destroyed by cooking; hence the value of eating fruits and vegetables raw. These foods

Enzymes naturally present in raw foods

Food	***Digests:***	**Sugars**	**Protein**	**Fat**	**Free radicals**
	Enzyme:	**Amylase**	**Protease**	**Lipase**	**Peroxidase Catalase**
Apple					•
Banana		•			
Cabbage		•			
Corn		•			
Egg (raw)		•	•	•	•
Grapes					•
Honey (raw)		•			•
Kidney beans		•	•		
Mango					•
Milk (raw)		•			•
Mushroom		•	•		•
Pineapple		•	•		
Rice		•			
Soya beans			•		
Sweet potato		•			
Wheat		•	•		

also need to be chewed properly, which helps to liberate and activate the enzymes they contain. The chart on page 17 shows those foods so far found to contain significant levels of health-promoting enzymes. This list, however, is far from complete, as many foods have not been investigated. Suffice to say that raw fruit and vegetables make a major contribution to our ability to digest, absorb and be nourished by our food.

In summary, you can improve your ability to digest food by following these enzyme-friendly steps:

- Take a digestive enzyme supplement with each main meal.
- Avoid over-eating. Eat little and often.
- Eat as much raw food as possible, chewing your food well.
- Choose enzyme-friendly foods, such as papaya, pineapple, sprouted beans and seeds, and fermented foods such as yoghurt.

CHAPTER 4

FOOD COMBINING – FACTS AND FICTION

Many people find that certain types or combinations of food don't suit them. Based on this observation and his research into health and nutrition, in the 1930s Dr Howard Hay devised a diet plan, popularly known as 'food combining', which has helped millions of people towards better health.

The key elements in Dr Hay's original theory were to eat 'alkaline-forming foods', avoid refined and heavily processed foods, eat fruit on its own, and not mix protein-rich and carbohydrate-rich foods.

As we have seen, protein and carbohydrate are digested differently. Carbohydrate digestion starts in the mouth when the digestive enzyme amylase, which is in the saliva, starts to interact with the food you chew. Once you swallow food and it enters the relatively acid environment of the stomach, amylase stops working. Only when the food leaves the stomach, where the digestive environment becomes more alkaline, can the next wave of amylase enzymes (this time secreted into the small intestine from the pancreas) complete the digestion of carbohydrate.

Protein, on the other hand, is not digested at all in the mouth. It needs the acid environment of the stomach and may hang around there for several hours until all the complex proteins are broken down into small groups of amino acids. This only happens in the stomach because of the high levels of hydrochloric acid which are needed to activate the protein-digesting enzyme, pepsin. Once small groups of amino acids leave the stomach, they meet peptidase enzymes (again from the pancreas) which break them down into amino acids, ready for absorption.

FOOD COMBINING MYTHS

The common, overly simplistic approach to food combining is to separate carbohydrate and protein foods because they are digested differently. The fact that eating certain kinds of beans produces flatulence is often quoted as a negative effect because beans are both protein and carbohydrate. However, it is now known that this is not the reason for beans' boisterous reputation. In some beans there are proteins, such as lectin, which cannot be digested by the enzymes in our digestive system, even when eaten alone. These proteins can, however, be digested by the bacteria that live in the large intestine. So when you eat beans you not only feed yourself, you also feed these bacteria. These bacteria produce gas after a good meal of lectin – hence the flatulence. It's got nothing to do with food combining. Many healthy cultures throughout the world have evolved to eat a diet in which beans or lentils are a staple food without suffering from digestive problems.

Protein and carbohydrate – foods that fight?

Of course, since foods aren't either exclusively carbohydrate or protein, in practical terms separating protein and carbohydrate actually means not combining *concentrated* protein foods with *concentrated* starch foods. Meat is 50 per cent protein/0 per cent carbohydrate. Potatoes are 8 per cent protein/90 per cent carbohydrate. In between are beans, lentils, rice, wheat and quinoa. So where exactly do we draw the line, if we draw a line at all?

THE EVOLUTION OF HUMAN DIGESTION

A brief excursion into our primitive past may solve the puzzle. The general consensus is that we, the human race, have been eating a predominantly vegetarian diet for millions of years, with the occasional helping of meat or fish. Monkeys can be divided into two types: those that have a ruminant-like digestive tract and slowly digest even the most indigestible fibrous foods, much like a cow; and those who have a much speedier and technologically advanced digestive system, producing a whole series of different enzyme secretions. We fit into the second category. The system is more efficient but can only handle foods that are easier to digest – fruit, young leaves, certain vegetables (no stalks for us!). Evolutionary theorists believe this 'latest model' digestive system did two things: first, it gave us the motivation to improve our mental and sensory processing so we would know when and where to find the food we needed; and second, it gave us the nutrients to make a more advanced brain and nervous system.

Did cavemen eat meat and two veg?

I believe we have three basic ways of digesting food. The first is for digesting concentrated protein (meat, fish and eggs). To digest these foods we have to produce vast amounts of stomach acid and protein-digesting enzymes. After all, if our ancestors had hunted down and killed an animal, do you think they then went off to pick a few tasty morsels of vegetation to create that 'balanced meal'? I doubt it. I imagine they ate their catch, organs and all, as fast as possible before it went off and other predators moved in. Perhaps they even had a couple of days on nothing but concentrated animal protein. Fresh, raw, organic meat is, after all, highly nutritious.

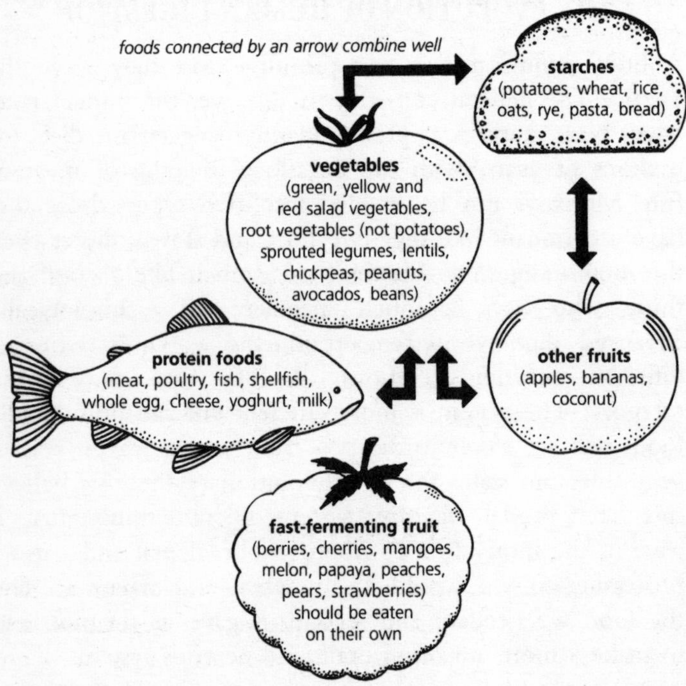

Figure 3 – Food combinations: dos and don'ts

Fruit – the lone ranger

At certain times of year we would have had access to certain fruits. No doubt we weren't the only fruit-eating creatures. Since fruit is basically the best fuel for instant energy, requiring very little digestion, we are good at producing the enzymes and hormones necessary to process its simple carbohydrates. Again, my guess is that we mainly ate fruit on its own. After all, once you've chomped your way through three bananas, you have little motivation to go digging up vegetables.

Many kinds of soft fruit ferment rapidly once they're ripe. They'll do the same if you stick them in a warm, acidic environment, which is what the stomach is. That's what happens if you eat steak and a melon in close succession. So Dr Hay's advice to eat fruit separately makes a lot of sense. Since fruit takes around 30 minutes to pass through the stomach, and concentrated protein takes two to three hours, this means that the best time to eat fruit is as a snack, more than 30 minutes before a meal, or not less than one to two hours after a meal, and possibly more if you eat a lot of concentrated protein. The only exception to this is combining fruits that don't readily ferment, like bananas, apples or pears, with complex carbohydrate-rich foods such as oats or millet. So apple porridge or a whole rye banana sandwich would be fine.

A HEALTHY BALANCE

However, most of the time, our ancestors seem to have eaten a varied vegan diet. That means leaf vegetables, root vegetables, nuts, seeds, pulses and sprouts. This, I propose, is the third and most common form of digestion – applied to a mixture of foods containing a mixture of carbohydrate and protein, but never as protein-dense as meat. I don't see any problem in combining rice, lentils, beans, vegetables, nuts and seeds.

While separating concentrated protein from concentrated carbohydrate may make digestion a little easier, it is now known that adding protein to a carbohydrate meal slows down the release of the sugars in carbohydrate, making it easier to keep your blood sugar level stable. This is particularly helpful as part of a weight loss strategy and for keeping energy levels even. Protein and carbohydrate separation may therefore be very beneficial for restoring proper digestion in those with enzyme deficiency, but is not necessarily a rule for life.

In a nutshell, food combining can be condensed into five simple steps (shown in Figure 3). If a person still has problems digesting these food combinations they may have a digestive enzyme deficiency, a food intolerance or dysbiosis, all of which are discussed in detail in this book.

In general, to give your digestion a helping hand:

- **Eat 80 per cent alkaline-forming foods and 20 per cent acid-forming foods.** This means eating large quantities of vegetables, fruit and lower protein foods like beans, lentils and wholegrains, instead of meat, fish, cheese and eggs.
- **Eat fast-fermenting and acid fruits on their own as snacks.** Most soft fruits ferment quickly. These include peaches, plums, mangoes, strawberries and melons. Highly acid fruits (although alkaline-forming) may also inhibit digestion of carbohydrate. This includes oranges, lemons, grapefruit and pineapple. All these fruits require little digestion, releasing their natural fructose content quickly. Eat them on their own as a snack when you need an energy boost.
- **Eat animal protein on its own or with vegetables.** Concentrated proteins (like meat, fish, hard cheese and eggs) require large amounts of stomach acid and a long stay in the stomach (around three hours) to be digested. So don't combine fast-releasing foods or food that ferments with animal protein.

- **Avoid all refined carbohydrates. Eat unrefined, fast-releasing carbohydrates with unrefined slow-releasing carbohydrates.** Fast-releasing fruits that don't readily ferment, such as bananas, apples and coconut, can be combined with slow-releasing carbohydrate cereals like oats and millet.
- **Don't eat until your body is wide awake.** Leave at least an hour between waking and eating. If you exercise in the morning eat after this. Never start your day with a stimulant (tea, coffee or a cigarette). The 'stress' state inhibits digestion. Eat only carbohydrate-based breakfasts such as cereal and fruit, just fruit, or wholegrain rye toast.

CHAPTER 5

PASSING THE ACID TEST

Although not an enzyme, one of the most critical factors in digestion is stomach acid. Too much or too little are common causes of digestive problems. Not only is stomach acid required for all protein digestion, it is also necessary for mineral absorption and is also your body's first line of defence against infections, effectively sterilising your food. So a lack of stomach acid (hydrochloric acid) leaves you unable to digest properly and prone to infections. This can lead to indigestion, particularly with high-protein meals, and the risk of developing food allergies because undigested large protein molecules are more likely to stimulate allergic reactions in the small intestine.

One of the most common reasons for a lack of stomach acid is zinc deficiency (because the production of hydrochloric acid is dependent on a sufficient intake of zinc). Hydrochloric acid production often declines in old age, as does zinc status. Estimates suggest that as much as half the population over the age of 60 suffers from hydrochloric acid deficiency.[2]

The symptoms of low stomach acid include burping after eating, bad breath, indigestion especially associated with protein-rich foods, upper abdominal pain, flatulence, bloating, diarrhoea or constipation. Another indicator is feeling full shortly after eating or the sensation that food is slow to pass from the stomach.

Stress also suppresses stomach acid production. This is because when we are stressed the body channels energy towards the 'fight or flight' response and away from digestion. So eating on the move or when you're stressed out is definitely a bad idea.

The nutritional solution to the problem of too little stomach acid is to take a digestive enzyme supplement containing betaine hydrochloride, plus at least 15mg of zinc in an easily absorbable form such as zinc citrate.

OVER-ACIDITY

Some people produce too much stomach acid, in which case supplementing betaine hydrochloride is likely to make matters worse rather than better. In most cases 'over-acidity' indicates that a person's stomach is having a hard time. When a baby eats something unsuitable the baby quickly vomits or gets diarrhoea. Continual dietary abuse hardens the stomach to such an immediate response but inflames and aggravates the stomach wall.

Alcohol, coffee, tea and aspirin all irritate the gut wall, as does an excessive intake of wheat products. Very hot drinks and spicy foods, especially chilli, are also stomach-unfriendly. Meat, fish, eggs and other concentrated proteins stimulate acid production. And this can aggravate the situation further because stomach acid will irritate an unhealthy and inflamed stomach lining that, when healthy, would produce its own protective mucous secretions. The conventional medical approach is to suppress the inflammation by giving a drug such as Tagamet (cimetadine). However, this doesn't deal with the underlying cause which is eating and drinking the wrong foods.

STOMACH ULCERS

The result of having a stomach-unfriendly diet is often stomach ulcers. Actually there are two kinds of ulcer –

peptic ulcers which are located in the stomach, and duodenal ulcers which are located just after the stomach in the duodenum. The simplistic view is that ulcers are due to excess stomach acid, but in fact the body is well designed to protect itself from its own healthy digestive juices. The trouble is that eating and drinking the wrong things damages the digestive tract which is then further aggravated by stomach acid. Cutting back on irritant foods and high-protein foods certainly helps reduce the immediate aggravation of existing ulcers but the ulcers still need to be healed.

Vitamin A is especially important for healing ulcers, while omega 3 fats (found in fish oils) help to calm down inflammation. Vitamin C, while helpful for healing ulcers, is a weak acid (ascorbic acid) and can therefore make matters worse. In fact, if you supplement vitamin C and experience fairly rapid gastric pain or burning it is well worth asking your doctor to check whether or not you have the early stages of an ulcer. Instead, supplement calcium or magnesium ascorbate (which are alkaline forms of vitamin C). What's more, the minerals calcium and magnesium are particularly alkaline and tend to have a calming effect on those suffering from excess acidity.

THE HELICOBACTER STORY

The majority of people with ulcers have been found to be infected with a bacteria called *Helicobacter pylori* which, unlike other bacteria, can survive in the high-acid environment of the stomach. Whether or not this bacterial infection is the original cause of digestive problems or the consequence of having an inflamed and aggravated digestive tract, there is little doubt that this infection makes matters much worse by reducing the body's production of protective gastric mucus, leading to inflammation and ulceration.[3] Being infected with Helicobacter increases a person's risk of having a duodenal ulcer by five times,[4] while 95 per cent of people with duodenal ulcers are infected.

Therefore anyone with ulceration, persistent indigestion or gastric pain is well advised to be tested for Helicobacter infection. This involves a simple blood test which your doctor can arrange for you. If the diagnosis is positive, conventional treatment involves specific antibiotics. There are, however, a wide range of natural alternatives which are discussed fully in Chapter 14.

HIATUS HERNIA

Another common cause of gastric pain and heartburn is having a hiatus hernia. Normally the stomach, which is located below the diaphragm muscle (see Figure 4), is closed off at either end by a circular muscle, thereby keeping the stomach acid contained. However, an estimated 50 per cent of people over the age of 50 have

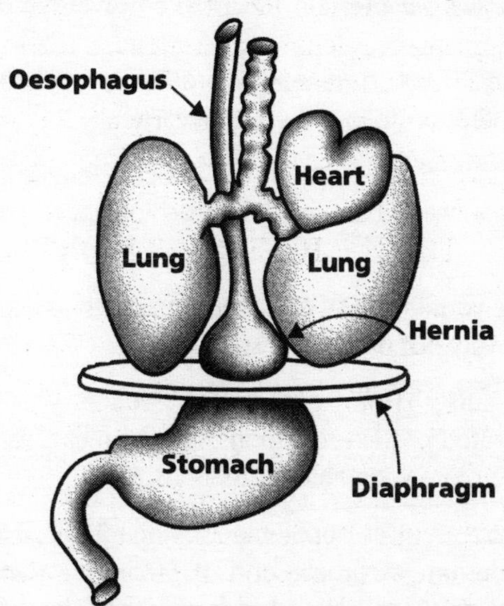

Figure 4 – Hiatus hernia

part of their stomach above the diaphragm muscle. This means that stomach acid can leak into the oesophagus, causing heartburn and gastric pain.

This physical defect, which can be relatively easily corrected, probably occurs for two reasons. The first is that the stomach can go into spasm when it is inflamed and irritated and may end up 'dislocated'. The other is a weakness in the diaphragm muscle (which is kept strong by deep breathing and exercise that stimulates deep breaths). Although it is said that having a genetically shorter oesophagus is a major cause, it is unlikely that this explains the prevalence of the problem. It is possible that an oesophagus in spasm could also pull the stomach up, again resulting in a hiatus hernia. In any event there are physical techniques practised by naturopaths and some osteopaths and kinesiologists that can help correct this condition. If muscle spasm is involved, capsules of peppermint oil, which is a muscle relaxant, can be beneficial (see Chapter 18 on irritable bowel syndrome).

In summary, if you have acidity problems, indigestion, gastric pain or ulceration follow these guidelines:

- If you have the symptoms of under-acidity supplement a digestive enzyme containing hydrochloric acid, plus 15mg of zinc.
- Minimise your intake of gastric irritants such as aspirin, coffee, alcohol, very hot drinks and spicy food.
- If you suffer from over-acidity reduce your intake of concentrated protein-rich foods such as meat, fish and eggs, and have more vegetable proteins instead.
- If you have an ulcer, supplement omega 3 fats, 1g of calcium or magnesium ascorbate and 10 000iu of vitamin A. You should also get yourself tested for *Helicobacter pylori*.

PART 2

IMPROVING ABSORPTION

CHAPTER 6

YOU ARE WHAT YOU ABSORB

It's one thing to completely digest your food and another thing to properly absorb it. The popular conception is that, once your food is digested, it just passes through the small intestine and into the body via the blood. In truth, there's much more to it than this. First of all, the small intestine isn't small. Although only about 6 metres in length, it has a surface area larger than a tennis court. The highly active cells that line this surface (the intestinal mucosa) are replaced on average every four days. If this surface area isn't healthy your ability to absorb nutrients from food and your ability to reject toxic substances won't be great either.

Different nutrients are absorbed through different sections of the small intestine (see Figure 5), each requiring a different set of conditions to maximise absorption. The duodenum, for example, is just one step down from the stomach, so it normally has a slightly acid environment which helps the absorption of minerals, fats and B vitamins. A lack of stomach acid, perhaps due to zinc deficiency, can have the knock-on effect of reducing the amount of nutrients absorbed (ironically, zinc itself can be affected by this). Vitamin B12 cannot be absorbed as such, but must first combine with a

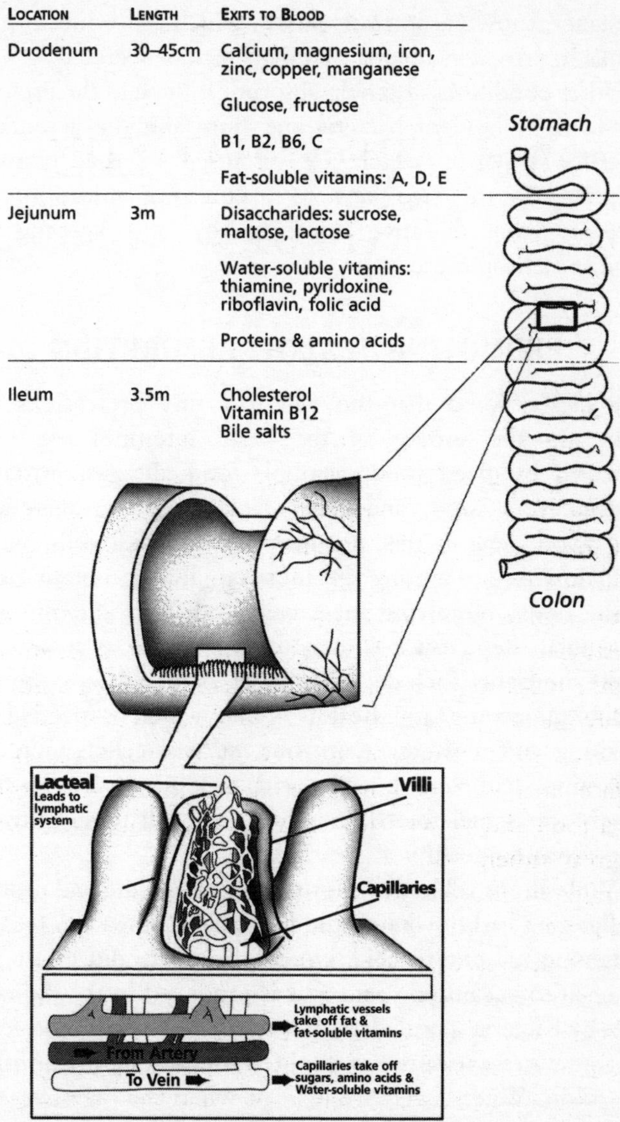

LOCATION	LENGTH	EXITS TO BLOOD
Duodenum	30–45cm	Calcium, magnesium, iron, zinc, copper, manganese Glucose, fructose B1, B2, B6, C Fat-soluble vitamins: A, D, E
Jejunum	3m	Disaccharides: sucrose, maltose, lactose Water-soluble vitamins: thiamine, pyridoxine, riboflavin, folic acid Proteins & amino acids
Ileum	3.5m	Cholesterol Vitamin B12 Bile salts

Figure 5 – Which nutrients are absorbed where and close-up of villi

substance known as intrinsic factor, which is produced in the stomach, provided adequate stomach acid is secreted.

Other conditions also help absorption, such as the presence of the right kind of bacteria and fibre and the absence of digestive irritants, which are discussed in the following chapters. So the two keys to maximising absorption are keeping your digestive tract healthy and keeping the environment in there just right.

PROMOTING HEALTHY ABSORPTION

The bad news is that the villi (the tiny protrusions that make up the surface of the small intestine) are easily damaged by fried food, alcohol, food allergies, irritating substances in food, and other factors such as infections. The good news is that the intestinal mucosal cells, which line the villi, are among the most rapidly regenerating cells in the body. Supplying these cells with the right nutrients is a vital step towards maximising nutrient absorption. These nutrients include: vitamin A, which keeps the cell membrane strong and healthy; zinc, which is needed for repairing and replacing worn-out mucosal cells; glutamine, an amino acid, and butyric acid, a kind of fat, both of which act as fuel for the mucosal cells. All these nutrients help promote healthy absorption.

While almost all body cells run on glucose (the end product of digesting carbohydrate), the intestinal mucosa can feed off glutamine and butyric acid. Under normal conditions there is no need to eat butyric acid as it is produced in the digestive tract by bacteria, particularly in the colon. Butyric acid levels are sometimes measured in stool tests to indicate the health of the colon. When levels are low, or when the digestive tract has become damaged and permeable, supplementing butyric acid can help restore digestive health (see Chapter 23). The same applies to the amino acid glutamine. While not an essential nutrient as such, it is certainly very helpful in nourishing, repairing and rebuilding the small intestine. It also strengthens immunity. Glutamine has also proven helpful for healing a damaged or permeable digestive tract, to aid recovery after surgery or after an infection.

If you have had a gastro-intestinal infection, or have been on antibiotics, or simply don't feel well nourished after a meal and suspect your absorption may not be up to scratch, you may benefit from supplementing 5–10g of glutamine. It is best, and generally much less expensive, to buy it as a powder. A heaped teaspoon is about 5g and should be taken with water, before going to bed. This is akin to feeding your lawn. As you sleep, glutamine helps your mucosal cells to regenerate and repair.

How absorption happens

While some nutrients simply pass into the body by diffusing across the intestinal wall, most are actively carried across by carrier molecules. These different absorption processes are themselves dependent on various nutrients, and cannot take place without them. So a vicious circle can arise if absorption of nutrients is under par, as the consequent lack of nutrients will further impair absorption. Glucose and amino acids are the nutrients which need to be actively transported across the intestinal wall and are therefore the most susceptible to malabsorption.

SETTING UP THE RIGHT CONDITIONS

Before food can be absorbed it must be prepared for absorption. This doesn't just involve digestive enzymes, it also involves enzymes that promote active absorption. These are dependent on nutrients – in other words, certain nutrients help other nutrients to be absorbed. An example is zinc and B6: this was demonstrated in an experiment in which animals were given increasing amounts of vitamin B6 and the same amount of zinc. The more B6 they were given, the more zinc they absorbed into the bloodstream.[1]

Some minerals, such as zinc and selenium, compete with each other for absorption, so, technically, they are better absorbed individually, on an empty stomach. However, unless you fancy swallowing supplements at several different times throughout the day, for practical purposes it is fine to do what nature does – take in nutrients as part of food. But bear in mind that certain foods contain substances that can interfere with the absorption of nutrients. These include:

- **Phytates** in wheat
- **Oxalates** in spinach and rhubarb
- **Methylxanthines** in tea, coffee, cocoa

The effect of these substances on the absorption of nutrients is not minor. For example, when you eat kale you absorb 40 per cent of the iron within it. However, when you eat spinach, which contain oxalates, you only absorb 5 per cent. Drinking a cup of coffee with a meal can also reduce iron absorption to a third.

Any substance that irritates the digestive tract, from alcohol to antibiotics, will also have undesirable effects on absorption. The chart opposite shows you what helps and what hinders your absorption of nutrients.

TESTING YOUR ABSORPTION

If your healthcare practitioner suspects you may not be absorbing properly they are likely to run one of two tests. The first is a stool analysis which can measure a number of factors that reflect your general ability to digest and absorb. These include the presence of proteins, fats and carbohydrates in the stool, indicating a compromised ability to digest and/or absorb your food.

Maximising absorption

FAT-SOLUBLE VITAMINS	Best form	When to take	What helps	What hinders
A	Retinol Beta-carotene	With foods that contain fat or oil	Zinc Vitamins E and C	Lack of bile
E	D-alpha tocopherol	With foods that contain fat or oil	Selenium Vitamin C	Lack of bile Ferric forms of iron Oxidised fats
D	Ergocalciferol Cholecalciferol	With foods that contain fat or oil	Calcium Phosphorous Vitamins E and C	Lack of bile

WATER-SOLUBLE VITAMINS	Best form	When to take	What helps	What hinders
B1	Thiamine	Alone or with meals	B complex Manganese	Alcohol Antibiotics Stress
B2	Riboflavin	Alone or with meals	B complex	Alcohol Antibiotics Smoking Stress
B3	Nicotinic acid Nicotinamide	Alone or with meals	B complex	Alcohol Antibiotics Stress
B5	Calcium pantothenate	Alone or with meals	Biotin Folic acid B complex	Antibiotics Stress
B6	Pyridoxine Hydrochloride + phosphate	Alone or with meals	Zinc Magnesium B complex	Alcohol Antibiotics Stress
B12	Cyanocobalamin Nasal gel	Alone or with meals	Calcium B complex	Alcohol Antibiotics Intestinal parasites Stress
Folic acid		Alone or with meals	Vitamin C B complex	Alcohol Antibiotics Stress

WATER-SOLUBLE VITAMINS	Best form	When to take	What helps	What hinders
Biotin		Alone or with meals	B complex	Antibiotics Avidin Stress
PABA	Para-amino benzoic acid	Alone or with meals	Folic acid B complex	Antibiotics Stress
Choline	Phosphatidyl Choline Lecithin	Alone or with meals	B5	Alcohol Antibiotics Stress
Inositol	Lecithin	Alone or with meals	Choline	Alcohol Antibiotics Stress
C	Ascorbic acid Calcium ascorbate	Alone, not with meals	Hydrochloride	Heavy meals

MINERALS	Best form	When to take	What helps	What hinders
Calcium	Chelate Carbonate Ascorbate	With protein food	Magnesium Vitamin D Hydrochloride	Tea/Coffee Smoking
Magnesium	Chelate Carbonate Citrate	With protein food	Calcium Vitamin B6 Vitamin D Hydrochloride	Alcohol Tea/Coffee Smoking
Iron	Ferrous forms Chelate Gluconate	With food	Vitamin C Hydrochloride	Oxalic acid Tea/Coffee Smoking
Zinc	Chelate Gluconate Orotate Sulphate	On empty stomach in the afternoon	Vitamin B6 Vitamin C Hydrochloride	Phytic acid Lead Copper Calcium Alcohol Tea/Coffee
Manganese	Chelate Gluconate Orotate	With protein food	Vitamin C Hydrochloride	High dosage of zinc Tea/Coffee Smoking
Chromium	Chelate Gluconate	With protein food	Vitamin B3 Hydrochloride	Tea/Coffee Smoking

MINERALS	Best form	When to take	What helps	What hinders
Selenium	Sodium selenite	On empty stomach	Vitamin E Hydrochloride	Coffee
	Selenium yeast	On empty stomach	Vitamin E Hydrochloride	Mercury Tea Smoking

A more specific indicator of absorption problems is an intestinal permeability test. Although there are different methods of determining intestinal permeability they all involve drinking something and then collecting a urine sample. This sample is then analysed to indicate what sizes of molecule are passing through the wall of your digestive tract. Therapeutic strategies for correcting identified absorption problems are outlined in Chapter 16.

In summary, unless you have an identified absorption problem, the following guidelines can help you maximise your ability to absorb nutrients from your food:

- If you drink tea, coffee or alcohol, don't have them with meals.
- Don't eat too much wheat.
- Supplement a high-strength multivitamin and mineral, giving at least 7500iu (2275mg) of vitamin A and 15mg of zinc, and take your supplements with food.
- Supplement 5g of glutamine before bed.

CHAPTER 7

THE FIBRE FACTOR

We all owe a lot to Dr Denis Burkitt and Dr Hubert Trowell who painstakingly travelled the world collecting stool samples. The conclusion of their research was that communities with loose-formed stools had very low incidence of colitis, diverticulitis, appendicitis, haemorrhoids and constipation, while communities with hardened, compacted stools were plagued by such digestive diseases, as well as the classic Western diseases of diabetes, heart disease and cancer. They identified the health-promoting ingredient as 'fibre'.

WHAT IS FIBRE?

Not all types of carbohydrate can be digested and broken down into glucose. Indigestible carbohydrate is called fibre. Fibre is a natural constituent of a healthy diet high in fruits, vegetables, lentils, beans and wholegrains. If you eat such a diet you have less risk of bowel cancer, diabetes or diverticular disease, and are unlikely to suffer from constipation.

Contrary to the popular image of fibre as mere 'roughage', it can actually absorb water. As it does so, it makes faecal matter bulkier, less dense and easier to pass along the digestive tract. This decreases the amount of time food waste spends inside the body and reduces the risk of infection or cell changes due to carcinogens that are produced when some foods, particularly meat, degrade. Bulkier faecal matter also means less chance of a blockage, or constipation.

There are many different kinds of fibre, some of which are proteins, not carbohydrates. Some fibre, such as that found in oats, is called 'soluble fibre' and combines with sugar molecules to slow down the absorption of carbohydrates. This type therefore helps to keep blood sugar levels balanced. Some fibre is much more water-absorbent than other types. While wheat fibre, for example, swells to ten times its original volume in water, glucomannan fibre (from the Japanese konjac plant) swells to 100 times its volume in water. Highly absorbent types of fibre, by bulking up foods and slowing down the release of sugars, can help to control appetite and play a part in weight maintenance.

HOW MUCH FIBRE?

The average daily intake of fibre in the UK and US is around 20g, which is less than half that of rural Africans who consume around 55g a day and suffer from few of the lower digestive diseases so common in the West. An ideal intake of fibre is not less than 35g a day. The chart overleaf shows you how much of each food you would need to eat to get 10g of fibre.

For example, if you have a cup of oats, an apple and a heaped tablespoon of seeds for breakfast this will provide 10g + 3g + 2g = 15g of fibre. A large salad containing crunchy vegetables, such as carrots, cabbage or broccoli pieces, may give you a further 15g. A meal based on beans, lentils or peas is likely to provide a further 15g.

Amount of food required to supply 10g of fibre

Food	Amount (for equivalent of 10g grain fibre)
All-Bran	37g/0.5 cup
Almonds	107g/0.8 cups
Apple	500g/3–4 apples
Apricots, dried	42g/1 cup
Baked beans	137g/small can
Baked potato (skin on)	400g/1 large
Bananas	625g/3 bananas
Broccoli	358g/1 large head
Cabbage	466g/1 medium
Carrots	310g/3 carrots
Cauliflower	475g/1 large
Coleslaw	400g/1 large serving
Cornflakes	91g/3.5 cups
Figs, dried	54g/0.3 cups
Lentils, cooked	270g/2 cups
New potatoes, boiled	500g/7 potatoes
Oatcakes	250g/10 biscuits
Oats	75g/1 cup
Oranges	415g/3 oranges
Peaches	625g/6 peaches
Peanuts	125g/1 cup
Peas	83g/1 cup
Prunes	146g/1 cup
Rice crispies	222g/8 cups
Rye bread	160g/6 slices
Sunflower seeds	147g/1 cup
Wheatbran	23g/0.5 cup
White bread	370g/15 slices
Wholemeal bread	115g/5 slices

Provided the right foods are eaten, 35g can easily be achieved without the need to add extra fibre. Professor of Nutrition, John Dickerson, from the University of Surrey, has stressed the danger of adding wheat bran to a nutrient-poor diet. The reason for this is that wheat bran contains high levels of phytate, which reduces the absorption of essential minerals, including zinc. Overall, it is probably best to get a mixture of fibre from oats, lentils, beans, seeds, fruits and raw or lightly cooked vegetables. Much of the fibre in vegetables is destroyed by cooking, so vegetables are best eaten crunchy.

TESTING GASTRO-INTESTINAL TRANSIT TIME

Apart from analysing what you eat, you can get a 'functional' indication of whether or not you're getting enough fibre by doing a very simple test to measure your gastro-intestinal transit time (the time it takes for food to pass through your digestive tract). Either buy some charcoal tablets and take 20 grains (or 1g), or eat a whole beetroot. Note the time and date you do this. When you see a darkened stool, in the case of the charcoal, or a reddened stool, in the case of the beetroot, you can calculate your transit time.

If your transit time is less than 12 hours you may not be absorbing all the nutrients from your food and you should investigate the possibility of absorption problems. If your transit time is more than 24 hours this indicates that waste material is spending too long inside you, a factor which increases your risk of colon-related diseases. This is a signal to increase your fibre intake and take some exercise which strengthens abdominal muscles.

Exercise helps because it promotes deeper breathing, so that the diaphragm (a dome-shaped muscle that separates the chest and abdominal cavity) is pulled down to allow for a deeper inhalation, and released as you exhale. This action massages the digestive tract and promotes bowel movements.

Drinking enough, water is also part of the equation. If you don't drink enough water the contents of your digestive tract are likely to become less watery and consequently harder to move along. The oils in ground seeds, such as flax seeds, also help to promote healthy bowel motions.

In summary, to keep everything moving along:

- Eat wholefoods – wholegrains, lentils, beans, nuts, seeds, fresh fruit and vegetables.
- Avoid refined, white, processed and overcooked foods.
- Exercise at least three times a week.
- Drink plenty of water – at least 1.5 litres a day.

CHAPTER 8

PROMOTING HEALTHY INTESTINAL FLORA

Did you know that up to 2kg of your body weight comes from bacteria? The average person has around 400 different types of friendly bacteria, mainly resident in the digestive tract, which are forever multiplying. There are about 100 trillion bacteria in your digestive tract, most of which are in the colon.[2] That's more than the total number of cells in your body. Every day you make quantities of bacteria and eliminate an equal amount in stools.

Not all of these bacteria are good for you, but, provided you have enough of the health-promoting bacteria, they act as your first line of defence against unfriendly bacteria and other disease-producing microbes including viruses and fungi. The good ones make some vitamins and digest fibre, allowing you to derive more nutrients from otherwise indigestible food, and also help promote a healthy digestive environment.

We are, in fact, partly descended from bacteria. Within our body cells are 'organelles' (or components), each with a specific function. Biologists now believe that the complex cells that make up our bodies may have developed from smaller micro-organisms, such as bacteria, 'working together'. Over time, this cooperation led to the development of the complex cells from which we are made. For example, the energy factories within our cells (called mitochondria) are derived from bacteria.

PROBIOTICS

So, the right kind of bacteria are our friends and are known as 'intestinal flora' or probiotics. The principal friendly bacteria include the families of Lactobacillus and Bifidus bacteria. The Bifidus family of bacteria generally makes up a quarter of the total flora in the digestive tract. Taking supplements of these friendly bacteria gives pathogenic (harmful) bacteria less chance of survival. There are many different strains of 'friendly' bacteria, some of which actually live in the gut, while others simply 'pass through' and are useful while they're there. Here are some of the different types:

The principal friendly bacteria

	Children	Adults
Resident	*B. infantis* *B. bifidum*	*L. acidophilus* *B. bacterium* *L. salivarius* *enterococci*
Passing through	*L. bulgaricus* *S. thermophilus*	*L. casei* (from cheese) *S. thermophilus* *L. salivarius* *L. bulgaricus*

Key: *B.* = *Bifidobacteria* *L.* = *Lactobacillus* *S.* = *Streptococcus*

Those that are resident, sometimes called 'human strain', are usually better at fighting infection because they multiply and colonise the digestive tract. Others are available in fermented foods, such as yoghurt, miso and sauerkraut. Yoghurt and other fermented dairy products often contain *Lactobacillus thermophilus* or *bulgaricus*. These bacteria will hang around for a week or so, doing good work. They, like the other beneficial bacteria, can make vitamins, as well as turning lactose (the main sugar in milk) into lactic acid. This makes the digestive tract slightly more acidic which inhibits disease-causing microbes such as *Candida albicans* from multiplying.

The benefits of having a healthy population of beneficial bacteria are many. They:

- **Make vitamins** including vitamins B1, B2, B3, B5, B6, B12, biotin, A and K.
- **Fight infections** and have been shown to halve recovery time from diarrhoea, prevent overgrowth of salmonella and *E.coli* (the bacteria responsible for many cases of food poisoning), *Helicobacter pylori* and *Candida albicans*.
- **Boost your immunity** by increasing the number of immune cells.
- **Promote other 'good' bacteria, while reducing 'bad' bacteria**. *Lactobacillus acidophilus* supplementation, for instance, has been shown to promote the beneficial bifidobacteria and inhibit disease-producing microbes.[3]
- **Repair and promote health of the digestive tract** because beneficial bacteria ferment sugars into short-chain fatty acids, such as butyric acid, which is used as fuel by the intestinal lining, helping it to repair itself.
- **Reduce inflammation** and have been shown to help conditions such as arthritis.[4]
- **Reduce allergic inflammatory reactions** by lessening the response in the gut to allergenic foods.[5] Many food reactions may not be solely due to food allergy but also due to the feeding of unfriendly bacteria which then produce substances that activate the immune system in the gut.[6]

PROMOTING HEALTHY BACTERIA

Many cultures have observed the health-promoting effects of fermented foods and include them as a regular part of their diet. These foods include:

- yoghurt, cottage cheese, kefir (from dairy produce)
- sauerkraut, pickles (from vegetables)
- miso, tofu, natto, tempeh, tamari, shoyu, soya yoghurt (from soya)
- sourdough bread (from wheat or rye, assuming you are not sensitive to wheat or gluten)

Including these foods in your diet is a good way to promote healthy intestinal flora. So too is eating foods that feed the intestinal flora. The best food for health-promoting bacteria is something called fructo-oligosaccharides (or FOS for short), which is sometimes known as a prebiotic. Bananas are especially rich in these, as are barley, fruit, garlic, Jerusalem artichokes, onions and soybeans. One study found that eating banana powder thickened the stomach lining, unlike aspirin which thins the stomach lining.[7]

Overall, eating a plant-based diet, high in fruits and vegetables, (which are naturally high in fibre), is much more likely to encourage healthy bacteria. On the other hand, a high-meat diet, apart from being the primary source of gastro-intestinal infections, is more likely to introduce toxic breakdown products as well as slowing down gastro-intestinal transit time.

RE-INOCULATING YOUR DIGESTIVE TRACT WITH PROBIOTICS

If you have had a major infection or have been treated with antibiotics you may benefit from a more direct way of 're-inoculating' your digestive tract by taking a probiotic supplement. The more 'broad-spectrum' the antibiotic, the more likely it is to devastate your colony of beneficial bacteria, leaving you even more susceptible to infection.

Healthfood stores stock probiotic supplements, many of which contain a combination of beneficial bacteria. The two most common families of bacteria provided are *Lactobacillus acidophilus* and bifidobacteria. Different strains are included according to whether the supplements are designed for children or adults, so you should seek advice on the best one to take, depending on your circumstances.

These supplements are made by culturing bacteria, then freeze-drying them. They are quite delicate organisms and are best kept in the fridge. When you swallow them and they come into contact with moisture, they come back to life. The best probiotic supplements also contain FOS for the bacteria to feed off, promoting their rapid multiplication, so check the label. FOS can also be supplemented on its own and has been shown to help promote more of the 'good guys' and reduce the 'bad guys', as well as relieving constipation.[8]

Generally, you need to take one or two capsules, or a teaspoon a day, providing around a billion of each strain of bacteria. It's best to take them with food if the bacteria are micro-encapsulated or enterically coated. Otherwise, take away from meals to minimise their destruction from gastric acid in the stomach. If you are taking probiotics therapeutically (for example, to re-inoculate the digestive tract after antibiotics or as part of an anti-infection strategy to kill off candidiasis), you may need three times this amount. These higher levels of probiotics and prebiotics such as FOS do sometimes result in increased flatulence, at least in the short term. This is not necessarily a bad sign. Sometimes, as less desirable organisms die off, symptoms get worse before they get better.

In summary, here are a few steps you can take to promote healthy intestinal flora:

- Eat a more plant-based diet.
- Eat fermented foods such as yoghurt, cottage cheese, miso, shoyu, sauerkraut and sourdough bread.
- Take a probiotic supplement containing beneficial strains of bacteria as well as FOS.

CHAPTER 9

Digestive Irritants – From Alcohol to Antibiotics

Many substances that we consume on a daily basis (quite apart from those foods that we are allergic to) are digestive irritants. These include alcohol, antibiotics, painkillers, certain spices, wheat, coffee and tea. In excess, these alone can be the cause of digestive problems.

ALCOHOL

Alcohol is an intestinal irritant, causing inflammation and damage to the digestive tract wall. This increases the risk of abnormal intestinal permeability, which, in turn, increases the likelihood of an allergic reaction, especially to the ingredients in the alcoholic drink. For this reason, about one in five beer and wine drinkers (on testing) show sensitivity to yeast. Wine drinkers become sensitive to sulphites, which are added to grapes to control their fermentation. Sulphites are also found in exhaust fumes; and the liver enzyme that detoxifies sulphites is dependent on molybdenum, a trace element which many people are deficient in. It's better to choose organic, sulphite-free wines and champagnes: and the latter has the added bonus of being yeast-free.

As well as increasing intestinal permeability, alcohol wreaks havoc on intestinal bacteria. It converts them into secondary metabolites that increase proliferation of cells in the colon, which can initiate cancer. It can also be absorbed directly into the mucosal cells that line the digestive tract, and converted into aldehyde which interferes with DNA repair and promotes tumours. In addition, some alcoholic drinks contain the carcinogen urethane. This is formed as a result of a chemical reaction that occurs during fermentation, baking or storage and has been found in American Bourbon whiskeys, European fruit brandies, cream sherries, port, saké and Chinese wine, but not vodka, gin or most beers.

According to the World Health Organisation, drinking alcohol has been linked to cancer of the throat, mouth, larynx, pharynx, oesophagus, bladder, breast and liver, with a substantially higher risk for those who smoke and drink. The World Cancer Research Fund reached the same conclusions and points out that the increased risk for colon and breast cancer occurs at very low levels of consumption. In the case of breast cancer a link starts to emerge above four drinks a week, while for colon cancer this association becomes stronger above a drink a day.

While there is a mildly protective effect from small amounts of red wine in relation to heart disease, overall regular alcohol consumption is very bad news for digestion and increases the risk of cancer. Specifically, it increases the risk of abnormal intestinal permeability and allergies and is therefore best avoided during any digestive health programme.

ANTIBIOTICS

Antibiotics are designed to kill bacteria and the more 'broad spectrum' an antibiotic is, the more it damages the vital, health-promoting bacteria in the digestive tract. What's more, the large quantity of antibiotic you need to consume to get enough into the bloodstream to fight, for instance, a sinus infection, creates a massive overload of antibiotics especially in the upper digestive tract. Since the intestinal flora protect the digestive tract, their destruction soon leads to inflammation and discomfort (experienced by most people taking antibiotics within 48 hours).

Antibiotics increase intestinal permeability and the risk and severity of allergies. For example, treating a child with an ear infection with antibiotics increases their risk of having another ear infection by five times. This is because ear infections are often the consequence of an allergy, often to dairy products, which results in excessive mucus production.

With the current global use of 50 000 tons of antibiotics each year, animals – including us – are becoming less resistant to disease, and bacteria are becoming more resistant to antibiotics. There is little doubt that this has played a part in the rapid escalation of food poisoning which now kills more than a million people a year worldwide.[9]

PAINKILLERS

The most commonly used painkillers, known as non-steroidal anti-inflammatory drugs (NSAIDs), are very bad news for digestion.

These include ibuprofen (Motrin), fenoprofen (Fenopron), flurbiprofen (Froben), ketoprofen (Alrheumat, Orudis and Oruvail), naproxen (Naprosyn), tolmetin (Tolectin), sulindac (Clinoril), azapropazone (Rheumox), indomethacin (Indocid), phenylbutazone (Butazolidine), mefenamic acid (Ponstan), diclofenac (Voltarol), fenbufen (Lederfen), piroxicam (Feldene), tiaprofenic acid (Surgam), as well as aspirin. In England alone, around 18 million prescriptions are written for these drugs each year.

The first drug that tends to be used to relieve pain and inflammation is aspirin; it can be quite effective but wreaks havoc on digestion. In 1980, the sixth World Nutrition Congress reported that even a single aspirin can cause intestinal bleeding for one week. Just imagine what high doses on a daily basis over many years are likely to do.

NSAIDs increase gut permeability[10] and ulcers in the small intestine, which can lead to serious complications. A study of athletes at the University of Iowa in the US, who took aspirin in order to prevent any inflammation, found that it significantly increased their intestinal permeability.[11]

A significant proportion of ulcers in the small intestine may be due to these drugs.[12] At least nine NSAIDs have been withdrawn from use, including Opren, and they are responsible for one quarter of all the reported adverse medication reactions. In the US the nation's spending on NSAIDs roughly equals the cost of treating the side-effects, many of which are gastro-intestinal reactions.

The chart opposite shows the percentage of people who experience gastro-intestinal problems from this class of drugs.

Acetaminophen (paracetamol) doesn't have the same irritant effect as NSAIDs but it is bad news for the liver. Gastro-intestinal irritation from painkillers overloads the liver's ability to detoxify (explained in Chapter 17), which is further compromised through use of this painkilling drug.

COFFEE AND TEA

Coffee contains a group of substances known as methylxanthines, including caffeine, theobromine and theophylline. These irritate the digestive tract and also bind to minerals, removing them before they are absorbed. So the consequences of drinking too much coffee are gastro-intestinal irritation and poor absorption of nutrients.

The same is true to an extent for tea. The chemicals present are somewhat different: tea has less caffeine but more tannin which binds to minerals and escorts them out of the body.

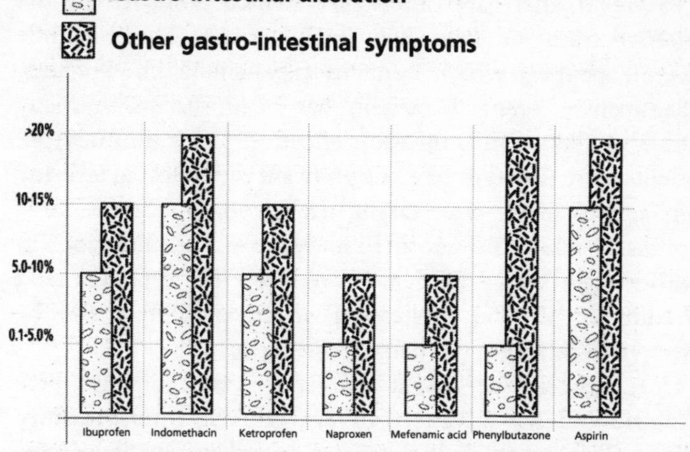

Figure 6 – Gastro-intestinal side-effects of long-term use of common painkillers

The odd cup of tea or coffee is unlikely to be a problem. However, anyone who is experiencing digestive problems, and has a regular, or excessive, intake of tea or coffee, is well advised to quit during a digestive healing programme.

Although herb and fruit teas don't contain gut irritants, any very hot drink is stressful on the digestive tract. The incidence of oesophageal cancer and stomach problems is higher among those who consume very hot drinks on a regular basis. So, it's best to avoid scaldingly hot drinks.

SPICES

Not all spices are created equal as far as digestion is concerned. Top of the 'bad' list is chilli. This acts as an intestinal irritant, especially in large amounts, and many people are actually quite allergic to it. If you don't react well to very 'hot' foods it is quite likely that you are allergic or sensitive to chilli.

However, there are other spices which don't irritate the digestive tract and may even be beneficial. These include cayenne pepper, which contains capsaicin, a known anti-inflammatory agent. Capsaicin has been shown in many studies to reduce inflammation effectively. In one study, 42 patients were found to have a significant reduction in arthritic pain and disability after taking these compounds for three months,[13] while in another study paw inflammation in arthritic rats was considerably reduced by capsaicin and curcumin.[14] Topical application of capsaicin may also be effective in relieving the pain of osteoarthritis.[15]

Curcumin is the bright yellow pigment of the spice turmeric and has a variety of powerful anti-inflammatory effects; trials in which it was given to arthritic patients have shown it to be roughly as effective as the anti-inflammatory drugs, without the side-effects.[16] It has also been shown to promote detoxification.

FIBRE AND ILEO-CAECAL VALVE PROBLEMS

While eating an unrefined diet, high in fibre, is generally good for you, some people experience a problem with certain kinds of fibre such as bran, and even raw foods. If this is true for you and you have inconsistent bowel movements – perhaps sometimes diarrhoea and other times constipation – then you may have a problem with your ileo-caecal valve. This is a circular valve-like muscle that separates the small intestine from the large intestine. It is located almost exactly midway between the right hip bone and tummy button. If this area is tender when you apply pressure to it, this is a further indication that you may have an inflamed ileo-caecal valve.

If the ileo-caecal valve doesn't open and close properly, or is too open, bacteria and toxins from the large intestine can move more easily than they should into the small intestine, leading to bacterial imbalance and self-intoxication. Proper ileo-caecal function can be disrupted by a diet that is too high in digestive irritants, including coarse fibres, or by constipation or loss of proper muscle tone and peristaltic muscle action that moves faecal matter along.

In such cases, the ileo-caecal valve function can be restored by two methods. One is a physical technique or manipulation practised by naturopaths, some nutritionists and kinesiologists. The other is by eating a diet that is very low in digestive irritants for a couple of weeks. This means excluding all the foods and drinks discussed in this chapter as well as wheat bran and any raw foods. Rather than adding fibre, or eating foods with added wheat fibre, which is very coarse, it is much better to obtain your fibre from wholefoods and, where applicable, soak them. For example, if you soak oat flakes to allow them to expand and absorb liquid, the fibres are much gentler on the digestive tract. Similarly, while raw food is good for almost everyone almost all the time, steaming or lightly cooking vegetables partially breaks down the coarser fibres.

In summary, if you want to be kind to your digestive tract:

- Avoid regular intake of tea, coffee and alcohol.
- Minimise your use of painkilling drugs, especially NSAIDs.
- Only consider antibiotics as a last resort, and, after a course of antibiotics, always take probiotics to restore your intestinal flora.
- Don't eat food spiced with chilli on a regular basis.
- Avoid added wheat bran; eat whole, unrefined foods instead.

CHAPTER 10

Our Deadly Bread

One of the most common intestinal irritants is wheat. Wheat is rich in a protein called gluten that contains gliadin which is known to irritate the intestines. A small amount may be tolerated, but many people consume wheat in the form of biscuits, toast, bread, cereals, cakes, pastry and pasta at least three times a day.

Modern wheat is much richer in gluten and hence in gliadin. This is because gluten, while bad news for your digestion, is good news for the baking industry. When yeast is fed sugar it produces gas. In the presence of the sticky protein gluten, this makes bubbles, and hence lighter loaves. This makes baked products look bigger and sell better. This kind of baking increases the amount of gluten available to react with the gut wall.

COELIAC DISEASE

While a high-gluten diet is bad news for anyone (as this sticky protein can clog up and irritate the digestive tract), some people are more severely sensitive to it. This is called coeliac disease, in which the tiny protrusions that make up the surface of the small intestine – the villi – get worn away. This results in various symptoms and malabsorption problems and a consequent loss of weight.

Coeliac disease is often undiagnosed as a cause of a variety of health problems including slow growth as a child and fatigue as an adult. A study involving 5000 high-school students in central Italy found that the prevalence of coeliac disease was close to one in every 200 students, with five in every six cases undiagnosed.[17] Coeliac disease leads to severe malabsorption of nutrients which can result in serious complications in later life, such as infertility, psychiatric disorders, osteoporosis and cancer. The condition does not always present with classical symptoms (including iron deficiency anaemia and short stature), which leaves many sufferers undiagnosed.

DIGESTIVE PROBLEMS AND WHEAT

However, you don't have to have coeliac disease to benefit from a wheat-free diet. A study at the Institute for Optimum Nutrition investigated the effects of removing wheat from the diet of 66 people who had digestive problems. They all craved bread and as a result ate a lot of it, not realising that wheat might be causing their digestive problems. During the study they abstained from eating wheat for a period of six weeks to investigate the possibility of food allergy or intolerance.

A total of 90 per cent experienced improvements in all their digestive symptoms; and 6 per cent had between 75 and 100 per cent improvement in all their symptoms. Six symptoms were reduced dramatically: constipation, flatulence, bloating, food cravings, lack of energy and mood swings. It is reasonable to suggest that these subjects were suffering from wheat intolerance.[18]

The most common symptoms of wheat sensitivity are constipation, diarrhoea, abdominal bloating or pain. However, many other symptoms have also been reported in those found to be sensitive to wheat. These include:

- nausea
- cramps
- flatulence
- fatigue
- throat trouble
- sweating
- skin rashes
- acne and boils
- migraine
- apathy and confusion
- depression
- anxiety and paranoia

INDIGESTION, GLUTEN SENSITIVITY OR WHEAT ALLERGY?

What isn't easy to establish is why these reactions occur. Since gluten is quite hard to digest, the suggestion is that too much of it is bad for anyone. Hence, everyone should eat fewer high-gluten foods, which essentially means fewer wheat products and especially wheat bread.

However, some people seem to react in a more allergic way, either to wheat or to all gluten-containing grains. If you appear to react to small amounts of wheat, or get non-digestive symptoms (such as feeling sleepy, anxious or depressed, or getting a headache) then you may have an allergy or sensitivity to either wheat or gluten. Ways of testing and treating such allergies are explained in the next chapter.

It is also possible, if you are allergic to wheat, that you may have become sensitive to all gluten grains. This is true in most people diagnosed with coeliac disease, in whom the best results are achieved by avoiding all sources of gluten. If you know you are allergic to wheat you may also wish to avoid spelt, which is an earlier type of wheat. (Although it contains less gluten, it may still cause you to react.) The grains which contain gluten (wheat being by far the most concentrated source) are shown below:

Gluten-containing grains	Gluten-free grains
Wheat	Corn (maize)
Rye	Rice
Oats	Quinoa
Spelt	Buckwheat
Barley	Gram (lentil flour)

Often, as part of a digestive healing programme, it is wise to go on a no-wheat, low-gluten diet for a month. Fortunately, there are many wheat-free and gluten-free options to choose from in healthfood shops and supermarkets these days:

- **Breads:** Rye bread, corn bread, rice cakes, oat cakes
- **Pasta:** Buckwheat spaghetti, soba noodles (buckwheat), rice noodles, quinoa pasta, corn pasta, polenta (maize)
- **Cereals:** Cornflakes, oatmeal, rice cereal, millet flakes.

THE PHYTATE CONNECTION

Provided you are not allergic to wheat or gluten and don't have a digestive problem, there is nothing wrong with eating grains. In fact, they are a good source of complex carbohydrate, fibre and other nutrients. However, if a large part of your diet is based on grains (bread, cereals, pasta, cakes, biscuits, etc), you may be eating too many phytates. A diet high in phytates, which are common components of various cereals, interferes with the absorption of many minerals including calcium.

A recent study has shown that this reduced absorption may have a considerable impact on bone density. Fourteen newly diagnosed adult coeliac patients were put on a gluten-free diet – which means they eliminated wheat, rye, oats and barley from their diet. After 12 months of gluten restriction, it was found that there was an overall increase in bone mass of 5 per cent in the lumbar spine and 5 per cent in the total skeleton. However, 11 of the 14 subjects, who followed the gluten restriction most strictly, had a greater increase in bone density – 8.4 per cent in the lumbar spine.[19] This study suggests that too many grains aren't good for anyone.

Generally speaking, to avoid these problems:

- Don't eat wheat every day; choose gluten-free or low-gluten grains instead.
- When you eat breads choose heavier, lower-gluten breads.
- Vary the grains you eat – have rye, oats, rice, barley, buckwheat, quinoa, corn.
- Limit grains to no more than a quarter of your total dietary intake.
- If you have a digestive problem or inflammatory bowel problem, investigate whether you are wheat- or gluten-sensitive.

CHAPTER 11

ALLERGIES – ONE MAN'S FOOD, ANOTHER MAN'S POISON

Food allergies and sensitivities are an almost inevitable consequence of problems with digestion and absorption. The body's immune system is highly active in the digestive tract and acts like a bouncer at the gateway into your body. If foods arrive at the gate undigested, or if the gate is damaged and inflamed, the ensuing chaos usually leads to some 'arrests' by the immune police. This is, in essence, what most food allergies or sensitivities are all about.

Of course, the real solution to allergies is to heal the digestive system and eat foods that don't stress or irritate the digestive tract. However, if you've already developed allergies, you first need to 'undevelop' them by finding out what foods you are currently allergic to and avoiding them long enough to heal the digestive tract and reprogramme the immune police.

ARE YOU ALLERGIC?

An estimated one in three people has an allergy. Some of these are to airborne substances such as pollen (hayfever),

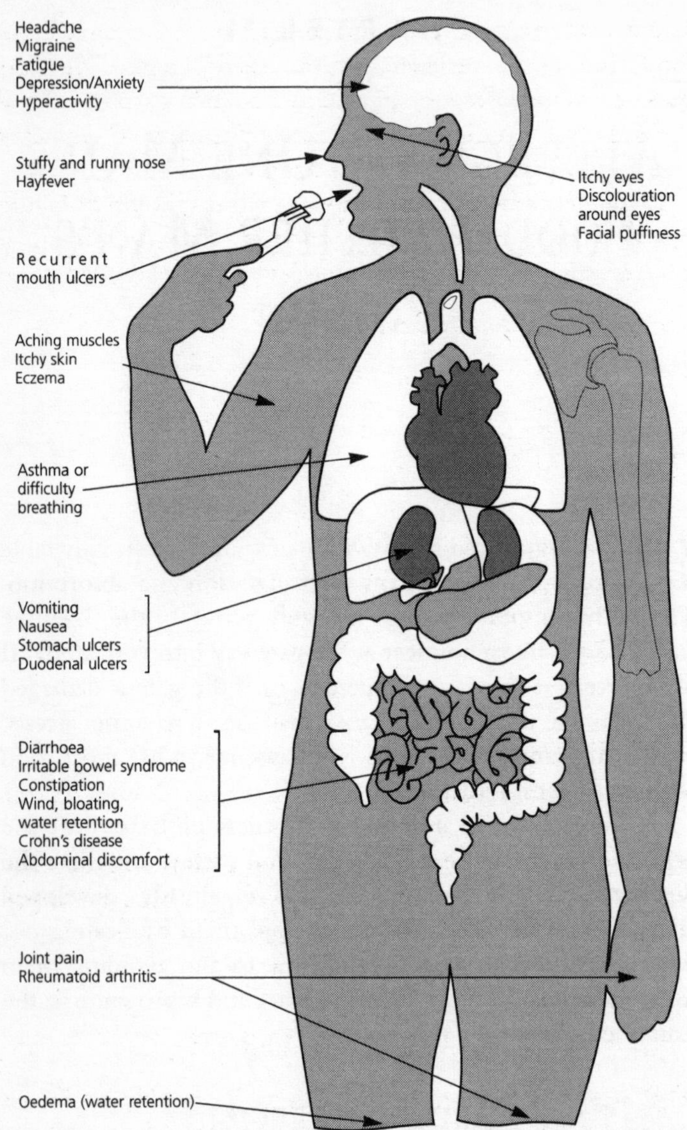

Figure 7 – Symptoms associated with food allergy and intolerance

house dust mite or cat's fur; others are to chemicals in food, household products or the environment. But the most common category of allergy-provoking substances is the food we eat. In a survey of 3300 adults 43 per cent said they experienced adverse reactions to food.[20]

If you get three or more of the symptoms shown in Figure 7, you probably have an allergy and most likely to something you are eating. The most common allergy-provoking foods are:

- wheat (bread, biscuits, cereals, pasta)
- dairy produce (milk, cheese, yoghurt)
- alcohol (especially beer and wine)
- coffee
- tea
- chocolate
- nuts
- eggs
- oranges
- chemical additives in food.

If you eat any one of these foods two or three times a day and would find them difficult to give up, it may be worth testing to see if you're allergic to them.

WHAT IS AN ALLERGY?

The classic definition of an allergy is 'any idiosyncratic reaction where the immune system is clearly involved'. The immune system (the body's defence system) can produce 'markers' for substances it doesn't like. The classic markers are antibodies called IgE (immunoglobulin type E). These attach themselves to 'mast cells' in the body. When the offending food (or allergen) combines with its specific IgE antibody, the IgE molecule triggers the mast cell to release granules containing histamine and other chemicals that cause the typical symptoms of allergy – skin rashes, hayfever, rhinitis, sinusitis, asthma, eczema. Severe allergies to shellfish or peanuts, for example, can cause immediate gastro-intestinal upsets or swelling in the face or throat. All these reactions are immediate, severe, inflammatory reactions and are known as Type 1 allergic reactions.

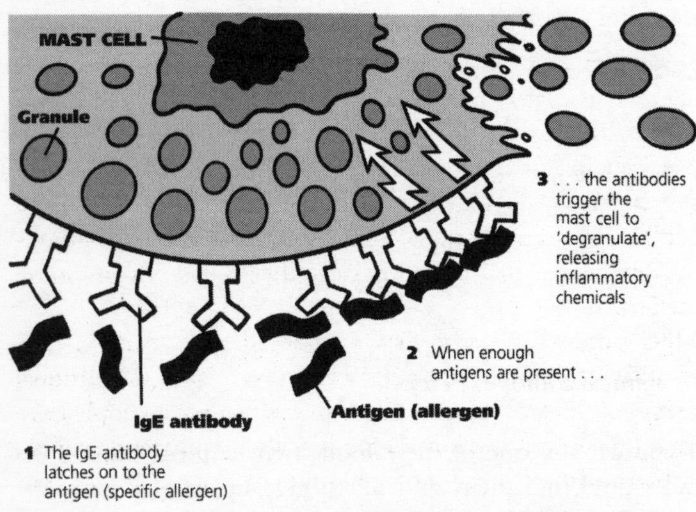

Figure 8 – How IgE-based allergic reactions happen

HIDDEN ALLERGIES

However, the emerging view is that most allergies and intolerances (diplomatically called 'idiosyncratic' reactions by some) are not IgE-based. There is a new school of thought and a new generation of allergy tests, designed to detect intolerances not based on IgE antibody reactions, but probably involving another marker, known as IgG. According to Dr James Braly, director of Immuno Laboratories, which developed the IgG ELISA test, 'Food allergy is not rare, nor are the effects limited to the air passages, the skin and digestive tract. Most food allergies are delayed reactions, taking anywhere from an hour to three days to show themselves, and are therefore much harder to detect. Delayed food allergy appears to be simply the inability of your digestive tract to prevent large quantities of partially digested and undigested food from entering the bloodstream.'

This is not a new idea. Since the 1950s, pioneering allergists such as Dr Theron Randolph, Herbert Rinkel, Dr Arthur Coca, and, more recently, Dr William Philpott and Dr Marshall Mandel, have written about delayed sensitivities having far-reaching effects on all systems of the body. These used to be the 'heretics' of classic allergy theory. But now their theories are being proved right, as scientific methods are developed for determining other types of immune reaction.

IgG antibodies were first discovered in the 1960s and are still considered rather irrelevant by some conventional allergists. The problem, say the critics, is that most people have many IgG-based reactions to foods without apparently suffering from allergies. The IgG antibodies may serve as 'tags' but they don't initiate a reaction. However, say the advocates, a large build-up of IgG antibodies to a particular food indicates a chronic, long-term sensitivity, or food intolerance. It is now well established that many, if not the majority, of food intolerances do not produce immediate symptoms, but have a delayed, cumulative effect. This, of course, makes them hard to detect by observation. Dr Hill, researching in Australia, found that the majority of food-sensitive children reacted to foods after two or more hours. In contrast, IgE reactions are immediate, suggesting that a build-up of IgG antibodies may be a primary factor in food sensitivity.

According to Dr Jonathan Brostoff, consultant in medical immunology at the Middlesex Hospital Medical School, certain ingested substances can cause the release of histamine and provoke classic allergic symptoms without involving IgE. These include lectins (in peanuts), shellfish, tomatoes, pork, alcohol, chocolate, pineapple, papaya, buckwheat, sunflower, mango and mustard. He also thinks it is possible that undigested proteins could directly affect mast cells (which contain histamine) in the gut, causing the classic symptoms of allergy.

One common cause of allergic reactions is a substantial production of antibodies (mainly IgG) in response to an allergen in the blood. This results in large immune complexes. 'It is the sheer weight of numbers that causes a problem,' says Brostoff. 'These immune complexes are like litter going round in the bloodstream.' The litter is cleaned up by cells, principally neutrophils, that act like vacuum cleaners. Cytotoxic allergy tests are designed to measure changes in number, size and activity of neutrophils when exposed to certain foods, to check for possible food allergies.

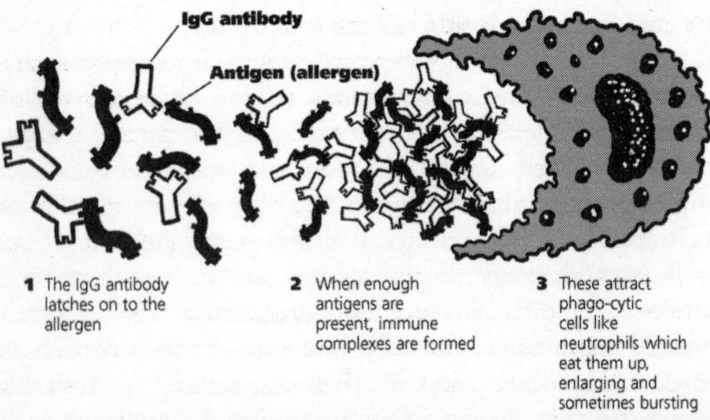

Figure 9 – How IgG-based allergic reactions happen

How IgG and IgE antibodies relate to one another is another area of debate. Allergy specialist Dr Braly has seen a number of patients who have both an immediate and a delayed reaction to a food, suggesting a link between the immediate IgE-type reaction and the delayed IgG reaction. Dr Anders Hoy from Denmark suspects that long-term build-up of IgG to a particular food might switch to an IgE-type sensitivity, causing immediate allergic response.

WHY FOOD ALLERGY?

Have you ever wondered whether the food you eat actually wants to be eaten? In most cases it appears that it does not. Most foods try their best to protect themselves from predators – with spikes, thorns and chemical toxins. The idea that food is 'good' is far from accurate. Most foods contain numerous toxins, as well as beneficial nutrients. Omnivores like us have a high risk–high return strategy as far as food is concerned. We try different foods and if we don't get sick then they're OK. But this short-term test can be dangerous. Indeed, even today, the average diet kills most people in the long run.

Some foods are designed to be eaten. For example, many fruits rely on animals eating them to spread the growth of their species. The idea is that animals, such as human beings, eat the fruit and deposit the seed some distance from the original tree with a rich manure starter kit. However, the fruit has to protect itself from unwanted scavengers such as bacteria or fungi that simply rot the seed. Seeds are therefore often hard to crack and toxic, such as apricot kernels which contain cyanide compounds. For these reasons, wild food contains a massive and often selective chemical arsenal to ward off specific foes. Food and us have been fighting for survival since the beginning of time.

So why do these food intolerances occur? Are they simply a reaction to less desirable toxins in our food? It is unlikely to be that simple. After all, we too have evolved over millions of years to protect ourselves from chemical poisons with complex detoxification processes which occur mainly in the liver. A number of theories exist, many of which have good supporting evidence.

Leaky gut syndrome?

The best place to start is the digestive tract since that is where food comes into contact with us. The textbooks tell us that large food molecules get broken down into simple amino acids, fatty acids and simple sugars. Only these get into the body. Anything larger is considered a foe. Could it be that undigested food, or leaky gut walls, could expose the immune system to food particles that trigger a reaction? This might explain why frequently eaten foods are more likely to cause a reaction. Indeed, recent research shows that people with food allergies do tend to have leaky gut walls (explained in detail in Chapter 16).

Dr Braly suspects that many allergy sufferers may have excessively leaky gut walls, allowing undigested proteins to enter the blood and cause reactions. Consumption of alcohol, frequent use of aspirin, deficiency in essential fatty acids or a gastro-intestinal infection or infestation (such as candidiasis) are all possible contributors to leaky gut syndrome. All these factors need to be corrected in order to reduce a person's sensitivity to foods. A lack of key nutrients, such as zinc, can also lead to weakening of the gut wall.

Gut-associated immune reactions

Although leaky gut syndrome may be part of the reason, it is unlikely to be the whole story. Evidence is accumulating to suggest that the gut wall is far less selective than originally thought, even in healthy people. In one study, healthy adults were given water containing potato starch – which should not normally pass across the gut wall intact. After 15–30 minutes blood samples contained up to 300 starch grains per millilitre of blood. So why aren't these people developing allergies?

This may be explained by special immune cells (known as Peyer's patches) which are present in areas along the digestive tract. These sample the food you eat and desensitise your immune system so that it doesn't react to your food. It seems that most food molecules are recognisably different from undesirable pathogens. Perhaps some people's gut-associated immune system isn't desensitising them to the food they eat. Indeed, their immune system may even be on red alert when certain food particles arrive. The result of this is that, as antibodies are released, they attach to the allergen-forming immune complexes and encourage inflammation. As well as leading to symptoms such as bloating, abdominal pain and diarrhoea, this may lead to undigested food passing through the gut wall, causing immune reactions in the bloodstream which then trigger symptoms that aren't specifically related to digestion.

Digestive enzymes

These problems may be particularly severe in people who don't produce enough of the right digestive enzymes, which means that large amounts of big, undigested food molecules reach the gut wall. One research study of people with a sensitivity to man-made chemicals showed that 90 per cent of them produced inadequate amounts of one digestive enzyme, compared with 20 per cent of healthy controls. Undigested food may increase the chances of a localised reaction, increase the amount of large molecules entering the blood, or simply provide food for undesirable bacteria in the gut, which then multiply prolifically. Often, taking digestive enzyme supplements reduces symptoms associated with food allergy and intolerance. Zinc supplements can also be helpful, as deficiency is extremely common among allergy sufferers. (Zinc is not only needed for protein digestion, it's also essential for the production of hydrochloric acid in the stomach).

Cross-reactions

Another contributor to food sensitivity is exposure to inhalants that provoke a reaction. For example, it is well known that, when the pollen count is high, more people suffer from hayfever in polluted areas than rural areas, despite the lower pollen counts in cities. It is thought that this is because exposure to exhaust fumes makes a pollen-allergic person more sensitive. Whether this is simply because their immune system is weakened from dealing with the pollution and therefore less able to cope with the additional pollen insult, or due to some kind of 'cross-reaction', is not known. In the US, where ragweed sensitivity is common, a cross-reaction with bananas has been reported. In other words, one sensitivity sensitises you to another. A similar cross-reaction may occur with pollen, wheat and milk for hayfever sufferers.

The emerging view, shared by an increasing number of allergy specialists, is that food sensitivity is a multi-factorial phenomenon, possibly involving poor nutrition, pollution, digestive problems and over-exposure to certain foods. Removing the foods may help the immune system to recover, but other factors also need to be dealt with in order to have a major impact on long-term food intolerance.

Food addiction

One interesting finding among people with food intolerances is that they often become hooked on the very food that causes a reaction. This can lead to bingeing on the foods that harm them most. Many patients describe these foods as leaving them feeling drugged or dopey. In some cases the foods induce a mild state of euphoria. In this way, the food can act as a psychological escape mechanism from uncomfortable situations. But why do some foods cause drug-like reactions? When pain no longer serves a purpose as part of a survival mechanism, chemicals called endorphins are released. These are the body's natural painkillers; they make you feel good. The way they do this is by binding to sites that turn off pain and turn on pleasant sensations. Opiates, such as morphine, are similar in chemical structure and bind to the same sites, which is why they suppress pain.

These endorphins, whether made by the body or taken as a drug, are peptides. Peptides are small groups of amino acids bound together – smaller than a protein and larger than an amino acid. When the protein that you eat is digested, it first becomes peptides and then, if digestion works well, single amino acids. In the laboratory, endorphin-like peptides have been made from wheat, milk, barley and corn using human digestive enzymes. These peptides have been shown to bind to endorphin receptor sites. Preliminary research does seem to show that certain foods, most commonly wheat and milk, may induce a short-term positive feeling, even if, in the long term, they are causing health problems.

Too often, the foods that don't suit you are the ones you 'couldn't live without'. This is exactly what happens in the case of many food allergies. If you stop eating the suspect food you may feel worse for a few days before you feel better. Some foods are addictive in their own right, such as sugar, alcohol, coffee, chocolate and tea (especially Earl Grey which contains bergamot). You can react to these foods without being allergic. Wheat, corn and milk could be added to this list on the basis of their endorphin-like effects.

REDUCING YOUR ALLERGIC POTENTIAL

A person can become food allergic for several possible reasons. Among these are lack of digestive enzymes, leaky gut, frequent exposure to foods containing irritant chemicals, immune deficiency leading to hypersensitivity of the immune system, micro-organism imbalance in the gut leading to leaky gut syndrome, and no doubt many more. Fortunately, tests exist to identify deficiencies in digestive enzymes, leaky gut syndrome, and the balance of bacteria and yeast in the gut. These tests are not available on the NHS, but can be arranged through nutritionists and nutritionally orientated doctors.

Apart from identifying and avoiding foods that cause a reaction, in order to allow the gut and immune system to calm down, there is a lot you can do to reduce your allergic potential.

For example, digestive enzyme complexes that help digest fat, protein and carbohydrate (lipase, amylase and protease) are well worth trying. Since stomach acid and protein-digesting enzymes rely on zinc and vitamin B6, it may help to take 15mg of zinc and 50mg of B6 twice a day, as well as a digestive enzyme with each meal.

Leaky guts can heal. Cell membranes are made out of fat-like compounds. And fatty acid – butyric acid – helps to heal the gut wall. The ideal daily dose is 1200mg. The essential fatty acids – linoleic and linolenic acid – are also important for maintaining proper gut permeability. Seeds (sesame, sunflower and pumpkin) are rich in these. The vitamin biotin, together with B6, zinc and magnesium, helps the body to use these fatty acids properly. Vitamin A is also crucial for the health of any mucous membrane including the gut wall. Supplementing these nutrients helps to heal a leaky gut – see Chapter 26 for recommended dosages. (Also see Chapter 16 for a more comprehensive strategy.)

Beneficial bacteria, such as *Lactobacillus acidophilus* or Bifidus, can also help to calm down a reactive digestive tract if the reaction is the result of a proliferation of the wrong kind of bacteria. If candidiasis is suspected, a different strategy is needed (see Chapter 15).

Boosting the immune system helps to reduce any hypersensitivity it may have.

HOW TO TEST FOR ALLERGIES AND INTOLERANCES

Of all the methods available for allergy testing, I believe the only reliable method is the elimination diet. If avoidance of a food leads to a reduction in symptoms and reintroduction leads to a worsening of symptoms then you know you have an intolerance to the food. It is worth checking the results of other tests by avoiding suspect foods and seeing if this makes a difference. The proof is in the eating, or rather the not eating.

Given that some foods may make you feel better in the short term and that some foods cause a delayed reaction, it is best to avoid all suspect foods for at least 14 days and preferably 30. If you don't know what you're reacting to you may get the best results by eating a very simple diet consisting of only foods with a low allergenic potential. The traditional elimination diet is lamb and pears. I prefer millet flakes, apple juice and apple for breakfast, with quinoa or rice plus vegetables for lunch and dinner. These diets are hard to follow for more than 14 days, as well as not being ideal nutritionally.

These are the steps you need to take:

1. Completely avoid the suspect food for 14 days.
2. On day 15 take your pulse at rest for 60 seconds.
3. Then eat more than usual of the food, e.g. three pieces of toast if you're avoiding wheat.
4. Take your pulse after 10, 30 and 60 minutes.

If your pulse goes up by 10 points, or if you have any noticeable symptoms within 48 hours, you probably have an allergy or intolerance to this food. The symptoms are more significant than the increased pulse, since some foods can raise the pulse without necessarily causing an allergic reaction. If you are testing more than one food and the first food caused a reaction, wait 48 hours before testing the next item. Otherwise reintroduce food number two the next day.

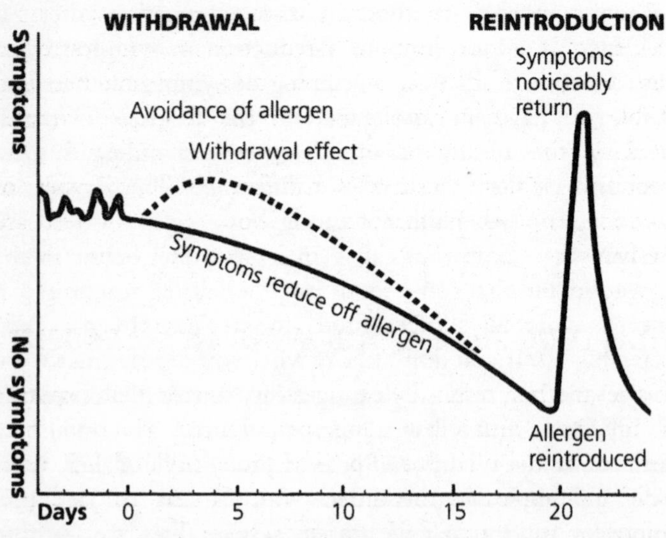

Figure 10 – The avoidance/reintroduction test for allergies

If you've ever had severe allergic reactions and/or an attack of asthma this test should not be carried out without the supervision of a doctor or nutritionist. If you suspect you have food allergies or intolerances I recommend you see an ION-trained nutritionist (see Useful Addresses) who can help you identify what you are reacting to and advise you on reducing your allergic potential.

Testing for IgG allergies

The first type of tests to move away from measuring immediate IgE reactions were the 'cytotoxic' (meaning 'toxic to cells') tests. These tests observe changes to immune cells called neutrophils which come along and clean up 'immune complexes' caused by antibody–antigen reactions. Cytotoxic tests are thought to indicate IgG sensitivity.

The state-of-the-art method for measuring IgG sensitivity is a relatively new technique, developed over the last eight years, known as ELISA. It claims more reproducible and reliable results than cytotoxic testing, and indeed samples tested by both methods have little agreement in results. One possibility is that these tests measure different types of reaction. Another is that one or both types of test are unreliable.

HOW LONG SHOULD YOU AVOID AN ALLERGEN?

This is another open-ended question. Foods that provoke an IgE-type, immediate and pronounced reaction may need to be avoided for life. The 'memory' of IgE antibodies is long-term. In contrast, B-cells that produce IgG antibodies have a half-life of six weeks. That means that there are half as many six weeks later. The 'memory' of these antibodies is short-term, and within six months there is not likely to be any residual 'memory' of reaction to a food that's been avoided. While a six-month avoidance may be ideal, Hoy and Braly report good results after as little as a month. Another option, after a strict one-month avoidance, is to 'rotate' foods so that an IgG-sensitive food is only eaten every four days. This reduces the build up of allergen-antibody complexes and reduces the chances of symptoms of intolerance. Foods such as wheat and milk which are, by their nature, difficult to digest, are probably best avoided as much as possible.

In summary, if you suspect you have allergies:

- Avoid suspect foods for 14 days and reintroduce them one by one, noting your symptoms; or have an allergy test.
- Avoid foods you test allergic to for three months while improving your diet to allow your digestive system to heal and desensitise.
- Reintroduce allergy-provoking foods one by one after three months, eating them infrequently, ideally no more than every four days, to minimise the chance of becoming allergic to the food once more.

PART 3

DIGESTIVE PROBLEMS AND SOLUTIONS

CHAPTER 12

THREE STEPS TO DIGESTIVE HEALTH

If you have followed the guidelines in Part 1 and Part 2 of this book, the chances are that your digestion is already much better and your digestive symptoms have been reduced. This is because most digestive problems are a consequence of one or more of the following:

- poor digestion (irritation, intoxication, lack of enzymes, lack of stomach acid)
- poor absorption (dysbiosis, increased gut permeability, allergies)
- poor elimination (clogged up colon, liver detoxification problems).

This common sequence of events is shown in Figure 11, together with the remedial actions necessary to get everything working properly again. These form the basis of the programme to restore digestive health, explained in more detail in Part 4.

The following chapters explore the most common digestive problems which affect almost everyone at some time in their lives. In fact, one survey found that almost 70 per cent

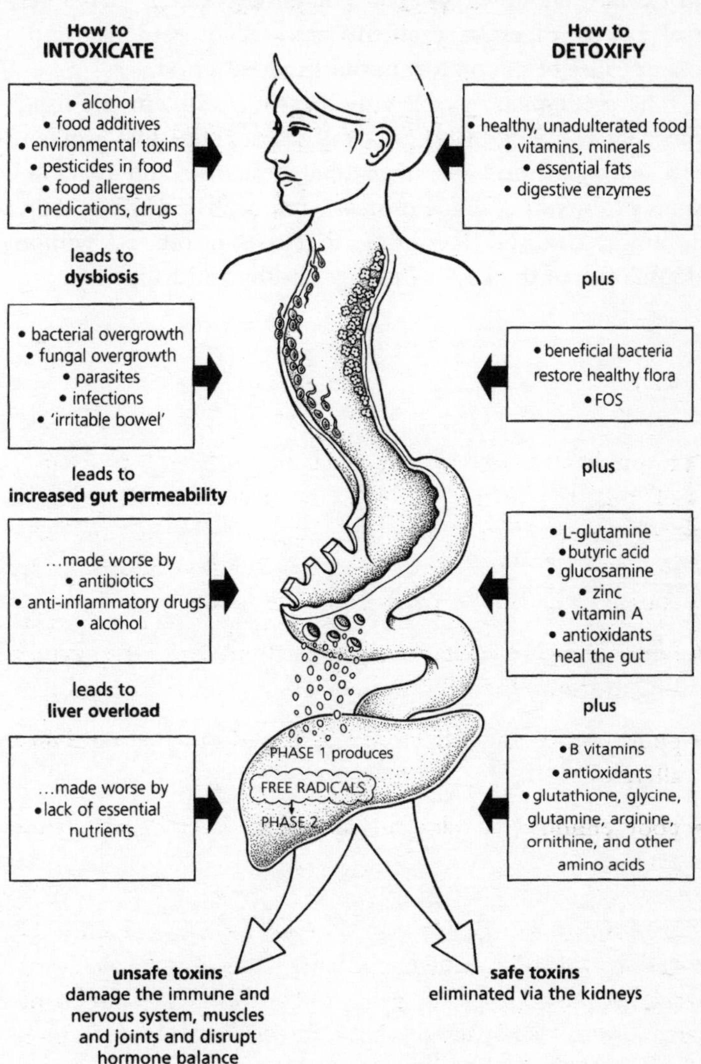

Figure 11 – What goes wrong, and how to correct it

of US households experience a digestive disorder.[1] To a very real extent, digestive problems are a silent epidemic and a major cause of discomfort in our modern world.

The consequences of having digestive problems are much more far-reaching than most of us realise. Digestive problems can lead to arthritis, chronic fatigue, headaches and migraines, sinus problems, eczema, psoriasis, infections and many other common diseases. Restoring digestive health is, without doubt, one of the keys to a long, healthy and happy life.

CHAPTER 13

Dysbiosis – When Things Go Wrong

When the balance of healthy bacteria in the digestive tract is disrupted and the 'bad guys' take over, this is called 'dysbiosis'. The term dysbiosis was coined at the beginning of this century by Dr Eli Metchnikoff, who succeeded Louis Pasteur as the director of the Pasteur Institute in Paris. He proposed that many digestive diseases resulted from an imbalance of micro-organisms in the digestive tract. Even though he won a Nobel Prize in 1908 for his work on the beneficial role of lactobacilli in boosting immunity, modern medicine essentially ignored his work in favour of producing antibiotics and other microbe-killing drugs. As a result, many disease-causing microbes have become resistant to drugs. These 'superbugs' now exist for staphylococcus and streptococcus infections, gonorrhoea, leprosy and tuberculosis. And many other bacteria have become resistant to specific types of antibiotic. Tens of thousands of people now die every year because no antibiotic can be found to treat their drug-resistant infections.

Understanding dysbiosis isn't about defining a new disease. Rather, it involves redefining the underlying cause of many diseases and reconsidering their method of treatment.

Virtually every disease discussed in this book has dysbiosis as an underlying root cause. Every chapter so far has introduced one factor after another that, if ignored, sets the scene for dysbiosis.

A lack of enzymes, too little stomach acid, vitamin and mineral deficiencies, eating allergenic food, exposure to disease-causing microbes, a lack of fibre, unhealthy intestinal flora – all these are the building blocks of dysbiosis. The symptoms are far-reaching because, once the digestive tract is no longer working properly, detoxification problems and inflammation are likely to follow.

Ironically, perhaps the greatest single contributors to dysbiosis are the very drugs used to treat the symptoms of these problems. Antibiotics, and steroid and non-steroidal anti-inflammatory drugs can all contribute to dysbiosis.

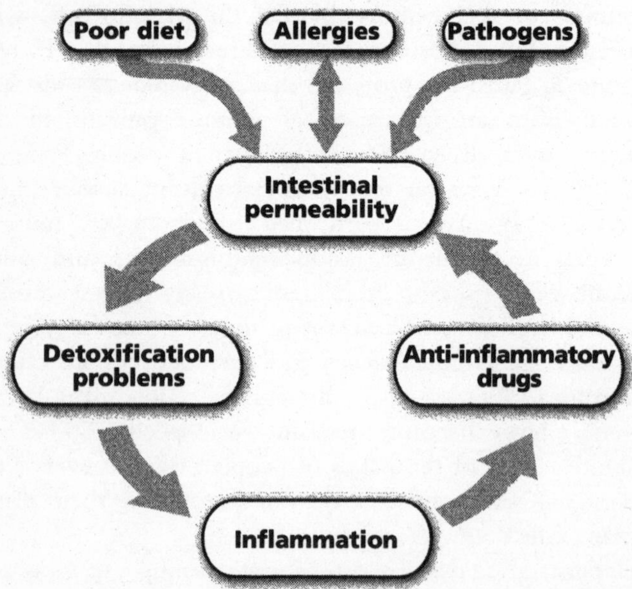

Figure 12 – The vicious circle of toxic overload

Steroid drugs feed Candida infections (see Chapter 15), while non-steroidal drugs are highly irritating to the digestive tract. Antibiotics, especially broad-spectrum antibiotics such as amoxycillin, not only wipe out the bad guys but also the good guys, removing our ability to keep further infections at bay.

The use of these drugs can generate the very conditions that lead to infection or inflammation, for which the conventional answer is more of the same drug. This may be good for business, but it's not good for your health.

Dysbiosis is about looking at the 'whole picture', the entire ecology of the digestive environment. According to Elizabeth Lipski, author of *Digestive Wellness*, there are four kinds of dysbiosis:

- **Putrefaction dysbiosis** – this is a consequence of food not being properly digested and eliminated, resulting in putrefaction and the generation of toxic by-products. The net result is bloating, discomfort and indigestion. This is the most common type of dysbiosis and the inevitable consequence of eating a high-fat, high-meat, low-fibre diet. This leads to too many of the bad guys (Bacteroides) and too few of the good guys (Bifidobacteria). The Bacteroides break down vitamin B12, so the person starts to experience deficiency symptoms such as fatigue, depression and weakness. They also convert bile into all sorts of toxins associated with promoting cancer.
- **Fermentation dysbiosis** – this is when the imbalance of micro-organisms favours those that ferment carbohydrate. Such people feel worse after eating carbohydrate or sugar-rich foods including fruit, beer, wine and grain products (such as bread or cereals).
- **Deficiency dysbiosis** – this occurs when a person is deficient in beneficial bacteria, perhaps as a result of a

course of antibiotics. Until their intestinal flora is returned to good health, they will be prone to irritable bowel syndrome, allergies and infections.

- **Sensitisation dysbiosis** – this occurs when the gut-associated immune system becomes highly sensitised to substances both in food and produced by microbes. Effectively, such a person becomes multi-allergic, and their symptoms are often systemic (i.e. not just in the gut). It is highly likely that many sufferers from auto-immune diseases, such as rheumatoid arthritis, lupus and possibly eczema and psoriasis, may fall into this category.

The solution is to find out exactly what's happening in a person's digestive ecosystem and then put it right. To this end, a clinical nutritionist is likely to recommend a 'comprehensive digestive stool analysis'. This can determine how well a person is digesting and absorbing and which of these four types of dysbiosis is present. For example, a high level of 'beta-glucoronidase' indicates putrefaction dysbiosis, while a high level of the yeast *Candida albicans* points to fermentation dysbiosis. An absence of sufficient lactobacilli or bifidus bacteria indicates a deficiency dysbiosis that may respond to supplementing these probiotic bacteria. Abnormal levels of immunoglobulin A (IgA) can indicate sensitisation dysbiosis and a greater risk of allergies. Such tests can also identify the presence of UFOs (unfriendly faecal organisms) which are the subject of the next chapter.

CHAPTER 14

UFOs OF THE INTESTINES

If you are experiencing diarrhoea and abdominal pain you may have been invaded by a UFO – an unfriendly faecal organism. As strange as it may sound, the presence of undesirable organisms (be they bacteria, viruses or parasites) in the digestive tract is surprisingly common. In under-developed countries up to 99 per cent of people have been found to house parasites, according to some surveys.[2] Diarrhoea-related diseases are some of the greatest worldwide causes of mortality. Although rarely life-threatening, such intestinal infections are probably present in one out of four people.

A recent UK survey estimates that nine million people a year experience some kind of stomach bug, and only one in every 136 infections is reported. However, many more people suffer insidious digestive symptoms which are rarely investigated. The frequency of world-wide travel is certainly one factor that has exposed more people to undesirable organisms. Many common parasites can also be encountered in water and improperly prepared food, or through poor hygiene practices and exposure to pets.

ARE UFOs YOUR PROBLEM?

While diarrhoea and abdominal pain are the two most common symptoms,[3] there are many other symptoms that may lead you to suspect that you have an intestinal infection. Consider the following ten questions:

1. Do you have chronic digestive symptoms?
2. Can you trace their origin to a trip abroad, swimming in a lake, a meal or any other event that may have inadvertently exposed you to an infection?
3. Is your abdomen distended no matter what you eat?
4. Do you almost always have dark circles under your eyes?
5. Do you get diarrhoea and irregular bowel motions?
6. Do you often experience abdominal pain?
7. Do your stools frequently smell foul?
8. Do you suffer a lot from flatulence?
9. Are you finding it difficult to maintain your weight?
10. Do you often feel worse after a meal?

If you answer 'yes' to the majority of these questions, it may well be worth investigating this area further.

Fortunately, tests for UFOs (generally known as 'parasitology tests') are not only becoming more precise but also more widely available and more frequently recommended by doctors. Having said that, I have found a great deal of disparity between laboratories, based on my own personal experience. Being a keen traveller, I spent a month in Tibet and the following year made two brief trips to Turkey and Morocco. After the initial trip to Tibet my digestion didn't seem to be as good as it used to be. I felt tired after meals, had discoloration under my eyes and slight nausea. I decided to find out if I had picked up any UFOs and also to 'test the tests'. So I sent off stool samples to Great Smokies Diagnostic Laboratory, one of the best laboratories in the US, and Parascope in the UK (see Useful Addresses), as well as going to my doctor. She referred me to a specialist who again ran a stool test for parasites. This showed nothing, while the former two laboratories both found high levels of two parasites. This is not uncommon since some NHS laboratories do not employ the latest techniques for identifying the presence of parasites. In 1976 a Newcastle study published in *The Lancet* showed that an adult with *Giardia lamblia* needed an average of 16 consecutive investigations before their parasitic infection was diagnosed.[4]

COMMON PARASITES

The two discovered in me were *Blastocystis hominis* and *Dientamoeba fragilis*. While there are literally hundreds of possible parasites, these are two of the 'top ten' found by parasitology laboratories. Parascope Laboratory, in Leeds, finds that some 40 per cent of specimens contain parasites. In the US, the Great Smokies Diagnostic Laboratory finds parasites in 20 per cent of samples tested. The Center for Disease Control (CDC) in Atlanta, Georgia, found that one in six randomly selected people had one or more parasites. Dr Hermann Bueno is one of the world's most experienced parasitologists, and he believes that 'Parasites are the missing diagnosis in the genesis of many chronic health problems, including diseases of the gastro-intestinal tract and endocrine system.'[5]

According to Antony Haynes, a clinical nutritionist specialising in the treatment of gut infections at The Nutrition Clinic in London, the following parasites are the most commonly identified in the UK:

- ***Blastocystis hominis*** – this is now widely considered to be a pathogen (a disease-causing organism). However, it is found in many people who have no symptoms, and should thus be treated only when symptoms are present. It can cause acute gastro-intestinal (GI) symptoms when present in large numbers or in weakened individuals, as well as irritable bowel, chronic fatigue, and arthritic and rheumatic complaints. It has been found in the synovial fluid in the

knee of an arthritis patient. It lodges within the intestinal lining, making eradication difficult.
Transmission: contaminated food, water and surfaces; surgery; tube feeding in hospital.

- ***Dientamoeba fragilis*** – infection can be asymptomatic, or present with diarrhoea and abdominal tenderness. There may be blood in the stool.
Transmission: contaminated water or swallowing pinworm eggs (food).

- ***Entamoeba coli*** – infection is often asymptomatic, but may be present with mild diarrhoea. The effects of the parasite infection go beyond digestive symptoms. Their presence can lead to the development of chronic 'all-over-the-body' symptoms.
Transmission: cysts from water or food.

- ***Giardia lamblia*** – these parasites stick to the upper part of the small intestine by means of a sucking disc, coating the lining of the intestine and preventing digestion and assimilation of food. A range of symptoms may be seen, including diarrhoea, constipation, malabsorption, fatigue, depression, bloatedness, flatulence, abdominal cramping, nausea and greasy stools. Whole towns and cities have been infected in recent history via contamination of the water supply (e.g. Aspen, Colorado, and St Petersburg, Russia).
Transmission: swallowing of cyst form which can be safely transported through the body, safe from destruction by digestive juices. It is at this stage that this parasite is infective because it may be transmitted by tap water or food infected with the cysts – via human or animal faeces – to another human.

- ***Endolimax nana*** – this is the smallest of a number of intestinal amoebas, and the most convincing research of its underestimated virulence comes from the British researcher

Dr Roger Wynburn-Mason. He suggests that *E. nana* is the cause of rheumatoid arthritis and a whole host of collagen-related diseases.[6] Some researchers believe that Wynburn-Mason may have misidentified the amoeba-like organism, although they agree that there is some kind of organism, to which many individuals have become genetically susceptible, which causes rheumatoid arthritis.
Transmission: tap water or contaminated foods.

Cryptosporidium – usually the infection is short-lived in healthy people, causing abdominal discomfort, weight loss, fever, diarrhoea and nausea. In those with weak immunity this parasite may result in much more severe problems because it can cause severe dehydration and electrolyte imbalances.
Transmission: contaminated ground water, farm animals, sexual contact and the faecal-oral route.

It is important to note, however, that the presence of some of these parasites doesn't necessarily mean a person will be unwell, or that they need treating. *Blastocystis hominis*, for example, is not always considered a pathogen, although there is increasing evidence that it can cause digestive problems in some people, according to Dr Ziertt at the US National Institute of Health.[7] One of America's medical experts in the treatment of parasites, he generally only recommends treatment if there is a positive test result and associated symptoms and especially if there is evidence of intestinal permeability (see Chapter 16). Due to the complexity of this area, if you suspect you have a problem it is important to consult a well-informed doctor or clinical nutritionist.

TREATING PARASITES AND OTHER UFOs

Conventional treatment of parasites, and indeed other UFOs – such as undesirable bacteria (including *Helicobacter pylori*, see Chapter 5) and yeasts (see Chapter 15) – involves a variety of antibiotic-type drugs with varying degrees of toxicity and capable of having damaging effects on beneficial intestinal bacteria. While these drug treatments may be necessary, especially for the most stubborn infections, they are often more effective if carried out alongside, or followed by, supplementation with less toxic natural remedies and probiotics. Some infections can be

Natural Remedy	Anti-bacterial	Anti-fungal	Anti-parasitic
Berberine (an extract from Goldenseal)	✓	✓	✓
Goldenseal	✓	✓	✓
Black walnut hull	✓	✓	✓
Oregon grape root extract	✓	✓	✓
Grapefruit seed extract (Citricidal)	✓	✓	✓
Echinacea angustifolia	✓	✓	✓
Garlic	✓		
Olive leaf extract	✓		
Pau d'arco		✓	
Quassia amara			✓
Chinese wormwood *(Artemesia annua)*	✓	✓	✓
Aloe vera	✓	✓	

swiftly treated with natural remedies without recourse to more toxic drugs. Your health practitioner can advise you on the best strategy. However, they are likely to employ one or more of the following natural remedies.

PREVENTING INFECTIONS

Prevention is better than cure and the best way to stay free of UFOs is to ensure that your immune system is fighting fit, your intestinal flora is flourishing, your digestive system is healthy and your exposure to potential UFOs is minimised.

The following habits can help reduce your risk:

- Drink filtered, distilled, bottled or boiled water, especially when abroad.
- Wash fruit and vegetables thoroughly.
- Wash your hands with soap before eating, and keep your fingernails short and clean.
- Cook food at the right temperature (above 180°F) to kill parasites and bacteria. Cook meat at 325°F or above, and bake fish at 400°F.
- Avoid raw foods such as sushi.
- Sanitise all toilet seats and bowls, especially those used by children.
- Don't walk barefoot, especially in warm moist, sandy soil.
- Don't use tap water to clean contact lenses. Use sterilised lens solutions.
- Keep toddlers away from puppies and kittens that have not been regularly wormed, and don't let them kiss animals.

CHAPTER 15

How to Beat Candida

One of the most common gastro-intestinal infections is called candidiasis. This is the overgrowth of the yeast-like fungus, *Candida albicans*. The name *Candida albicans* means 'sweet and white', suggesting something delicate and pure. But, in reality, *Candida albicans* is a minute microbe, a yeast, which multiplies, migrates and releases toxins. It can afflict us with countless symptoms (bowel problems, allergies, hormone dysfunction, skin complaints, joint and muscle pain, thrush, infections and emotional disorders), many of which mimic other diseases and are frequently misdiagnosed.

People who suffer from this microbe often personify Candida as an enemy, against whom they must wage long and determined war. The only certain path to victory is to understand its tactics and take the offensive with all guns blazing. This enemy will lose no opportunity to regain lost ground, so the battle must be unrelenting until at last it is won – and even then there is the danger of a false treaty.

Yet this distressing situation is largely of our own making. We eat a lot of refined sugar which yeast loves; antibiotics used indiscriminately reduce friendly bacteria and create more room in the intestines for pathogenic microbes; steroid drugs and hormone treatments depress the immune system so that it cannot fight off pathogens effectively; and the formulas in babies' bottles ensure an early imbalance in bowel ecology.

Candida cannot take all the blame; we give it every encouragement. The first stage in fighting back is therefore to start taking responsibility for our health.

Obviously, it is important to ensure that the enemy is correctly identified. Dr William Crook published a questionnaire in his book, *The Yeast Connection*, which can help ascertain the presence or severity of an overgrowth of Candida. If it shows a high score and if doctors have failed to make any other diagnosis, it makes sense to embark on an anti-Candida campaign, with the support of a clinical nutritionist.

THE CANDIDA QUESTIONNAIRE

Answer the questions below, ticking those that you answer 'yes' to.

History	**yes**
Have you taken tetracycline or other antibiotics for one month or longer?	☐
Have you, at any time in your life, taken other 'broad-spectrum' antibiotics for respiratory, urinary or other infections (for two months or longer, or in shorter courses four or more times in a one-year period)?	☐
Have you, at any time in your life, been bothered by persistent prostatitis, vaginitis or other problems affecting your reproductive organs?	☐
Have you taken birth control pills for more than two years?	☐
Have you taken cortisone-type drugs for more than a month?	☐
Does exposure to perfumes, insecticides, cigarette smoke and other chemicals provoke noticeable symptoms?	☐

History	**yes**
Are your symptoms worse on damp, muggy days or in mouldy places?	☐
Do you have athlete's foot, ring worm, 'jock itch' or other chronic fungal infections of the skin or nails?	☐
Do you crave sugar, bread or alcoholic beverages?	☐

Score 2 points for each 'yes' answer

Symptoms	**yes**
Do you often experience fatigue or lethargy?	☐
Do you ever feel 'drained'?	☐
Do you suffer from depression?	☐
Do you have poor memory?	☐
Do you ever feel 'spacey' or 'unreal'?	☐
Do you suffer from an inability to make decisions?	☐
Do you experience numbness, burning or tingling?	☐
Do you ever get headaches or migraines?	☐
Do you suffer from muscle aches?	☐
Do you have muscle weakness or paralysis?	☐
Do you have pain and/or swelling in your joints?	☐
Do you suffer from abdominal pain?	☐
Do you get constipation and/or diarrhoea?	☐
Do you suffer from bloating, belching or intestinal gas?	☐
Do you have troublesome vaginal burning, itching or discharge?	☐
Do you suffer from prostatitis or impotence?	☐
Do you ever experience a loss of sexual desire or feeling?	☐
Do you suffer from endometriosis or infertility?	☐
Do you have cramps or other menstrual irregularities?	☐
Do you get premenstrual tension?	☐

Symptoms	**yes**
Do you ever have attacks of anxiety or crying?	☐
Do you suffer from cold hands or feet and/or chilliness?	☐
Do you get shaky or irritable when hungry?	☐

Score 1 point for each 'yes' answer

Add up your total score. If you score above 30 there's a strong likelihood that you have candidiasis. If you score above 20 there's a possibility that you have a degree of candidiasis. We recommend you see a nutrition consultant and have appropriate tests to find out if candidiasis is your problem.

THE ANTI-CANDIDA FOUR-POINT PLAN

1. Diet

The aim of this diet is to starve the Candida. As sugar encourages fungal growth, it must be strictly avoided in all its forms, including lactose (milk sugar), malt and fructose (fruit sugar). Refined carbohydrates add to the glucose load so it is essential to use only wholegrain flour, rice, etc. Other substances to be avoided are yeast (bread, gravy mixes, spreads), fermented products (alcohol, vinegar), mould (cheese, mushrooms), and stimulants (tea, coffee). A positive approach to the diet is essential, and we recommend that you read the *Beat Candida Cookbook* by Erica White to show that mealtimes can still be an enjoyable experience!

Candida often brings on cravings for its favourite foods; at these times steely determination is needed to keep to the diet. Motivation is encouraged by a clear understanding of what is happening. Even when Candida-related symptoms have completely disappeared, the diet should be maintained for a further year to consolidate the newly corrected balance of gut flora. Before long, a 'sweet tooth' disappears, making it easier to stay on a sugar-free diet.

2. Personal supplement programme

A supplement programme can help correct imbalances in glucose tolerance, hormonal status and histamine level, and can also help detoxify the body of pollutants. It is important to support the immune system in as many ways as possible in order to fight back against Candida. The situation should be monitored and the programme reassessed at three-monthly intervals.

In an otherwise carefully calculated programme of nutrients devised by your nutritionist, Vitamin C may be taken to bowel tolerance levels to help rid the body of toxins. In addition, pantothenic acid (vitamin B5), 500mg, twice a day, may further reduce the adverse effects of these toxins.

3. Anti-fungal supplements

One of the most useful anti-fungal agents is caprylic acid, a fatty acid which occurs naturally in coconuts. Its great advantage is that it does not adversely affect beneficial organisms. It is fat-soluble, so will penetrate cell membranes. As calcium/magnesium caprylate, it survives digestive processes and is able to reach the colon. For reasons yet to be discussed, it is essential to start with a low level and build up slowly, a process facilitated by different-strength capsules (see page 101).

Artemesia is a herb with broad-spectrum anti-fungal properties, useful against a wide variety of pathogens without disturbing friendly microbes. A high score on the Candida questionnaire and a history of illness originating in a hot climate are sufficient reasons to suspect a parasite other than Candida, and to use a broad-spectrum anti-fungal agent.

Propolis is another natural substance which, according to research at the University of Bratislava, is remarkably effective for all fungal infections of the skin and body. It can be taken as drops and built up gradually. Its anaesthetic effect is soothing for oral thrush, and, as cream, for painful muscles.

Aloe vera is gently anti-fungal and is a refreshing mouthwash or gargle as well as an ingestible aid to digestion. It can also be used as an overnight denture soak (preferable to products which are not specifically anti-fungal). Dentures can be an ongoing source of Candida re-infection.

Tea tree oil is an anti-fungal agent and, as a cream, can be used for fungal skin conditions. Candida is frequently associated with eczema, psoriasis and acne, as well as athlete's foot and other fungal skin or nail infections.

Grapefruit seed extract, also called Citricidal, is a powerful antibiotic, anti-fungal and anti-viral agent. The great advantage, however, is that it doesn't have much effect on the beneficial gut bacteria. It comes in drops, best taken two or three times a day, 15 drops at a time, and in capsules. Other anti-fungal preparations include oregano oil, olive leaf, garlic, goldenseal and pau d'arco.

With gentle experimentation, the most suitable natural anti-fungals can soon be discovered. Consult a nutritionist or herbalist to determine the best dosage levels for your particular digestive problem.

4. Probiotics

Supplements are needed to carry beneficial bacteria into the intestines and re-establish a healthy colony. The Americans call it 're-florestation'! The role of these Bifidobacteria is to increase acidity by producing lactic acid and acetic acid, and to inhibit undesirable micro-organisms that would compete against them for attachment sites. Tissues densely covered with beneficial organisms provide an effective blocking mechanism, deterring invading pathogens.

Lactobacillus acidophilus is the major coloniser of the small intestine and *Bifidobacterium bifidum* inhabits the large intestine and vagina; it also produces B vitamins. Other helpful bacteria are the transient *Lactobacillus bulgaricus* and *Streptococcus thermophilus*, which also produce lactic acid as they pass through the bowel. These friendly bacteria are contained in yoghurt which is therefore a helpful food, provided there is no intolerance to dairy foods (although you could try live goat's milk or sheep's milk yoghurt if it's only cow's milk you are sensitive to). In yoghurt, the lactose (milk sugar) content has largely been converted into lactic acid by enzyme-producing Bifidobacteria, which accounts for the sharpness of its taste.

To ensure that these bacteria travel safely through the gastric juices, you need to take them in a capsules supplying large numbers of viable organisms in freeze-dried form. Two capsules should be taken daily, at breakfast and supper, but this may be increased to six daily or even more in cases of diarrhoea or of illness necessitating antibiotics (which further deplete the Bifidobacteria). An acidophilus cream is a beneficial aid for a vaginal fungal infection.

Each of the points in this four-point plan is essential in the fight against Candida. Non-compliance with any one of them may lead to failure. There is also a fifth vital aspect – support. Anyone entering this 'war zone' will experience confusion and depression. Someone is needed who can look at the situation objectively, discern what is happening and point the way forward. This is part of the role of an effective nutritionist.

DEALING WITH DIE-OFF

Thriving Candida releases a minimum of 79 known toxins. Dead Candida releases even more. A general feeling of toxicity includes aching muscles, fuzzy head, depression, anxiety, nausea and diarrhoea. In specific areas where Candida has colonised, there will be an apparent flare-up of old symptoms – sore throat, thrush, painful joints, eczema, etc. This unpleasant situation is known as 'die-off' (or, formally, as Herxheimer's reaction). It has to be recognised as a last-ditch deception by the enemy because the very presence of the symptoms means that Candida is being wiped out and that victory is imminent.

The art is to destroy Candida slowly but surely so that it is not being killed off faster than the body can eliminate the toxins. Initial die-off is usually triggered by the diet, as Candida is starved, and by vitamins and minerals as they boost the immune system to fight it. These first two points of the four-point plan usually cause more than enough die-off for most people to cope with, and anti-fungal agents should not be added to the regime until this phase is over. By the end of a month the majority of people claim that they feel better than they have for years! Then is the time to add caprylic acid and acidophilus supplements to the programme.

Taking ground slowly is still the surest method of attack. Most people on caprylic acid can start by tolerating one medium-strength 400mg capsule daily, without too much difficulty. If, after five days, they are not battling with die-off symptoms, the dose can be increased to two 400mg capsules, and so on up to six capsules daily. After this, they can graduate to three 680mg capsules, and increase again if necessary. However, progress is seldom straightforward and at some stage there might come a surge of die-off reaction, necessitating a drop to a lower level, or even a complete break, whilst the body eliminates the toxins. This should not be regarded as a setback, but simply as a necessary part of the process. Drinking plenty of fluid and taking good levels of vitamin C and pantothenic acid, as already discussed, will speed up detoxification. Eventually, caprylic acid does its job and the score on the Candida questionnaire falls to as low as it can, allowing for 'history' factors which obviously do not change.

Slow progress might be due to environmental factors (e.g. domestic gas or mould from house-plant soil) or food sensitivities overloading the immune system. Avoidance of culprit foods once identified through pulse-testing (see Chapter 11) enables the immune system to work more efficiently. Discovering environmental culprits involves detection and possibly expense if, for instance, the heating system needs to be changed!

Candidiasis is frequently not acknowledged by medical practitioners and can be misunderstood by family and friends. Loneliness and despair add to the physical and mental suffering created by the enemy within. There is no easy way to win the Candida war. It takes courage, determination and perseverance – but it can be done.

CHAPTER 16

LEAKY GUT SYNDROME

Normally healthy foods can also become toxins to the body if they are not digested or absorbed properly. We are designed to digest our food into simple molecules that can readily pass through the digestive tract and into the bloodstream. If, however, a person doesn't digest their food properly, or if the gut wall becomes leaky, incompletely digested foods can enter the blood. There they are likely to alert immune 'scout' cells which treat them as invaders, triggering an allergic reaction. The ensuing battle results in a complex of chemicals that are themselves toxic and need to be cleaned up.

The integrity of the gut wall is therefore critical to our health and our bodies work hard to maintain its proper permeability in the face of considerable 'assault' on a daily basis. It is now recognised that this permeability, while remarkable in its complexity, is vulnerable and subject to change, depending on the integrity of the gut wall and the substances it is exposed to. Increased permeability, far from enhancing the transport of nutrients, allows the entrance of toxins and improperly digested food particles which can give rise to a number of health problems associated with 'leaky gut syndrome'.[8]

Symptoms and conditions associated with leaky gut syndrome

- acne
- AIDS/HIV infection
- arthritis (osteo-/rheumatoid)
- autism
- childhood hyperactivity
- chronic fatigue syndrome
- chronic hepatitis
- chronic pancreatitis
- coeliac disease
- cystic fibrosis
- depression, mood swings
- diarrhoea/constipation
- eczema
- fatigue
- food/chemical sensitivities
- inflammatory bowel disease (Crohn's, ulcerative colitis)
- irritable bowel syndrome
- psoriasis, dermatitis
- urticaria (hives)
- viral, bacterial or yeast infection

The lining of the digestive tract is a remarkably complex 'skin' which performs countless functions – digesting foods, absorbing them, moving food along, providing immune protection and so on. Its folds, lined with villi, perform the seemingly contradictory task of acting as both a barrier to toxins and large food particles and a one-way, selective gate to nutrients. This careful balance is confronted every day by a host of toxins and allergens, which – with optimum health of the mucous membranes, proper permeability, immunity, liver function and flora – pose no danger. If, however, any of these are compromised, ill-health is likely to follow.

Because this highly selective permeability of the intestine makes it so vulnerable to bad dietary habits and bacterial imbalances, it has developed several complex protection mechanisms.

Nutrients are transported across the gut lining in one of two ways: either through the cells themselves (transcellularly); or through the gaps, or 'tight junctions', between the cells (paracellularly) as shown in Figure 13. When either or both of

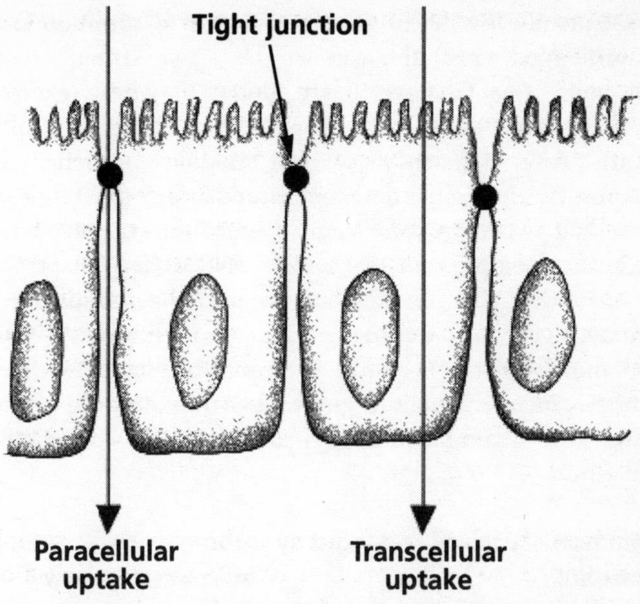

Figure 13 – How nutrients pass across the gut lining

these mechanisms become faulty the gut becomes increasingly permeable, or 'leaky', allowing unwanted substances to pass across the gut wall. The gut wall is protected by intestinal secretions which consist of, among other substances, protective mucus, immune cells that act as a benevolent police force, and secretory IgA. This is an immunoglobulin that acts like the bouncer in a nightclub. Each IgA molecule can remember what should or shouldn't pass into the body, and whistles up immune cells to get rid of unwanted guests. If IgA levels are very low this natural protection is lost.

WHAT CAUSES INCREASED PERMEABILITY?

The intestinal tract can become leaky for a number of reasons. If a person's immune system is weakened, with consequently low levels of secretory IgA (a common factor in prolonged stress) this can set the scene. Irritants to the gut lining (see Chapter 9) are gluten in wheat, excessive alcohol, coffee, tea and many other allergy-provoking foods. Any deficiency of cell-building nutrients, like vitamin A, zinc, glutamine and essential fats, can result in a poor gut wall structure. An overgrowth of the wrong bacteria or fungi, such as *Candida albicans* (see Chapter 15) or any other parasite, can burrow into the intestinal wall, irritating it and causing increased permeability. Even abdominal distention, either as a result of bloating or over-eating, can overstress the gut wall. Antibiotics, aspirin and other anti-inflammatory drugs are especially damaging to the gut.

Common causes of leaky gut syndrome

- alcohol
- antibiotics
- anti-inflammatory drugs (e.g. aspirin)
- chemotherapy/radiotherapy
- dysbiosis (bacterial imbalance)
- food allergies
- gastro-intestinal disease
- infections (bacteria, viruses, yeasts, parasites)
- inflammatory bowel disease
- long-term stress
- low-fibre diet
- nutritional deficiencies (e.g. vitamin A, zinc, glutamine, omega 3 essential fats, etc)
- poor digestion
- secretory IgA deficiency

As we have seen, increased permeability does not increase the absorption of essential nutrients. Indeed, this is likely to be reduced, as the workings of the lining are affected by damage and inflammation. Once gut permeability is increased, a vicious circle may begin, whereby the passage of toxins and undigested food particles into the body creates conditions which further exacerbate the situation:

liver overload, malabsorption, allergy (see Chapter 11) and dysbiosis (see Chapter 13).

LEAKY GUT – CONSEQUENCES OR CAUSES?

Ironically, once the liver becomes increasingly overloaded with toxins (see Chapter 17) toxic chemicals can be excreted in bile and re-enter the digestive tract, hence contributing to further intestinal damage.[9] Also, the increased inflammation of the digestive tract actually stops the body absorbing health-promoting nutrients needed by the liver and by the body to produce digestive enzymes. It's a vicious circle in which leaky gut syndrome creates the conditions for leaky gut syndrome![10]

The link between allergies and a leaky gut is another 'chicken-and-the egg' situation in that each can give rise to the other. Allergies may manifest in a number of ways, including eczema, fatigue, etc. Some scientists propose that food allergies contribute to leaky gut syndrome in asthmatics due to an increased allergy load overwhelming the gut's immune system.[11] Dr Leo Galland, author of *The Power of Healing*, suggests that chemicals such as histamine, released in response to allergens, increase permeability. A number of studies have shown that people with food allergies have increased permeability in a fasting state which is further exacerbated when an offending food is ingested.[12]

Dysbiosis (an imbalance of gut flora) is also a likely cause and consequence of leaky gut syndrome. A low level of stomach acid can contribute, since this normally destroys micro-organisms that can further damage the digestive tract. It appears that increased permeability can even lead to the gut's immune system over-reacting to normal gut bacteria as well as pathogenic organisms, once again increasing permeability.

ASSESSING GUT PERMEABILITY

In view of the fact that leaky gut has been implicated in an array of health problems, restoring the condition of the intestinal lining may be a key factor in improving digestive health. If you have any of the health problems listed on page 104 that have not responded to treatment, or if you score high on the list of common causes on page 106, it would be well worth your while finding out if you have increased intestinal permeability.

There are tests that can give a clear indication of how leaky (or permeable) the gut lining is. This is done by drinking certain chemicals that are not digested in the human body and then taking a urine sample to measure how readily they have passed through the intestinal wall. Small molecules (e.g. mannitol) easily diffuse through cells, while larger molecules (e.g. disaccharide lactulose) do not normally pass across the intestinal wall. Mannitol can therefore be used to measure absorption through cells and lactulose acts as a marker for the integrity of the gaps between cells (tight junctions). So a gut permeability test involves the ingestion of particular amounts of these two molecules in a solution. Urine gathered over the next six hours is then checked for its levels of mannitol and lactulose and compared with a pre-test sample.

High levels of lactulose in the post-ingestion urine sample show that there is increased intestinal permeability or a 'leaky gut', while low levels of mannitol indicate that malabsorption of nutrients is a problem. A clinical nutritionist would be able to arrange such a test and interpret the results.

HEALING A LEAKY GUT

Healing a leaky gut broadly involves three steps:

1. remove the cause

2. improve gut flora and function
3. repair the gut

In order for the cause of leaky gut to be removed, it must first be detected. Factors to consider are drugs (such as NSAIDs), alcohol, caffeine, allergy-provoking foods, UFOs, Candida overgrowth or dysbiosis. Any improvement in intestinal health is unlikely while these are still present.

Meanwhile it is essential to provide the gut with an ample supply of the nutrients needed for good health and repair, such as vitamin A, zinc, glutamine, essential fatty acids, antioxidants, n-acetyl-glucosamine and fibre.

The presence of friendly bacteria in adequate numbers is also crucial in developing and sustaining a healthy gut. Probiotic supplements containing a range of bacteria including various lactobacilli and Bifidus species can help this, especially when given alongside FOS (fructo-oligosaccharides). It is important to ensure good digestion: from proper chewing and adequate levels of stomach acid to sufficient output of digestive enzymes. Each of these may be taken as supplements.

At the same time, you should avoid suspected allergens (usually wheat, gluten and dairy products), sugar, refined carbohydrates, saturated fat and meat; and have plenty of water, fibre, and water- and nutrient-dense whole foods.

CHAPTER 17

Liver Detoxification Problems – The Cause of Chronic Fatigue?

If you have increased intestinal permeability your liver will be working overtime to deal with the extra toxins, improperly digested foods and potential allergens that can get through your digestive tract into your blood. A good 80 per cent of the chemical processes that go on in the body involve detoxifying thousands of potentially harmful substances. Much of this is done by the liver which represents a clearing house, able to recognise millions of potentially harmful chemicals and transform them into something harmless or prepare them for elimination. It assembles amino acids, stores vitamins and minerals, makes cholesterol and bile, controls glucose and fat supplies, balances hormones and plays a key role in immunity. It is the chemical brain of the body – recycling, regenerating and detoxifying in order to maintain your health.

Most of us tend to assume that food is always good for us. Of course it is, but the truth is that almost all food contains toxins as well as nutrients. So too do air and water. These external or exo-toxins are just a small part of what the liver has to deal with; many toxins are made by the body from otherwise harmless molecules. Every thought, every breath and every action generate toxins. These internally created or endo-toxins have to be disarmed in just the same way as exo-toxins. Whether a substance is bad for you or not depends as much on your ability to detoxify it as on its inherent toxic properties. People with multiple food sensitivities are eating the same food as healthy people – they have just lost their ability to detoxify it.

Instead of thinking of certain substances as 'bad' for you, or provoking allergies, think of them as exceeding your adaptive capacity. It's as if the body's metabolism represents a fire. The fire generates smoke that needs to be got rid of. Our metabolic fire (the consequence of using the energy from the sun stored in plants) burns slowly and generates plenty of smoke. That's what the liver has to deal with. It's the 'smoke', not the substances themselves, that often causes problems.

DETOXIFICATION – A TWO-STEP PROCESS

The way the liver detoxifies this smoke can be split into two stages. Phase 1 is akin to getting your rubbish ready for collection. It doesn't actually eliminate anything, just prepares it for elimination, making it easier to pick up. Fat-soluble toxins, for example, become more soluble. Phase 1 is carried out by a series of enzymes called P-450 enzymes. The more toxins you're exposed to, the faster these enzymes must work to pile up rubbish ready for collection. Often, the substances created by the P-450 enzyme reactions are more toxic than before. For example, many are oxidised, generating harmful free radicals.

The function of P-450 enzymes depends on a long list of nutrients, including vitamins B2, B3, B6, B12, folic acid, glutathione, amino acids (leucine, isoleucine, valine), flavonoids and phospholipids, plus a generous supply of antioxidant nutrients to deal with the oxidants. A person who has a high exposure to toxins (due to diet and lifestyle

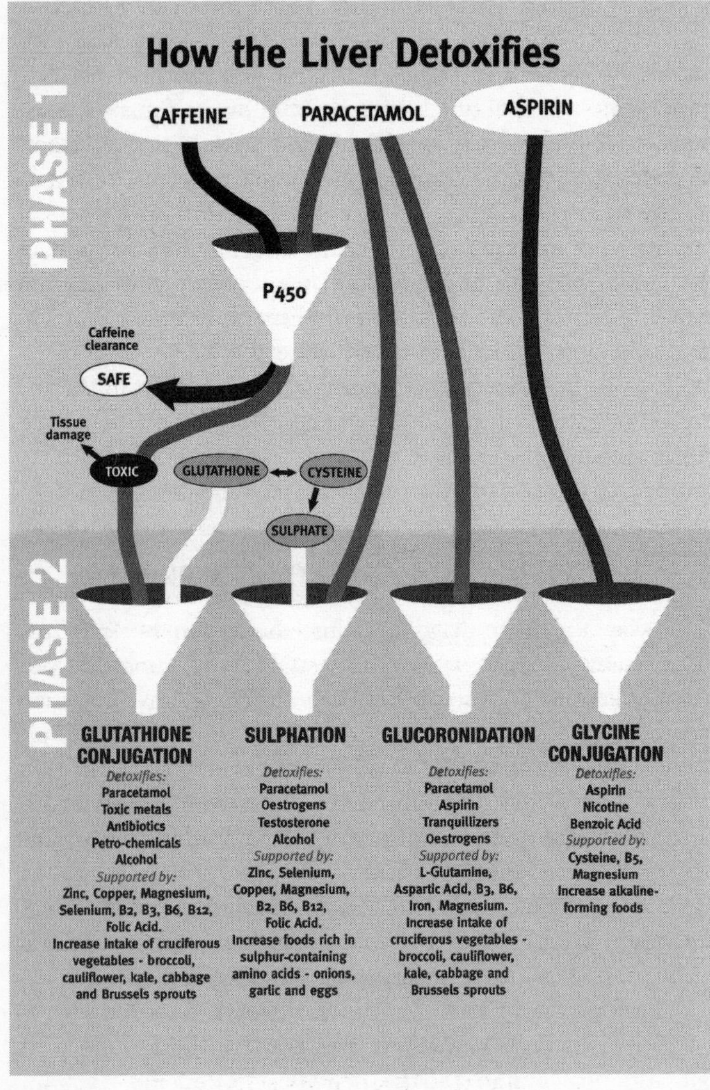

Figure 14 – How the liver detoxifies

factors or digestive problems) may have a revved up Phase 1, used to working hard and fast to get these toxins ready for collection. Substances that get Phase 1 going include caffeine, alcohol, dioxins, cigarette smoke, exhaust fumes, high-protein diets, organophosphate fertilisers, paint fumes, saturated fat, steroid hormones and charcoal barbecued meat.

The next stage, Phase 2, is more about building up than breaking down. According to Dr Sidney Baker, an expert in the chemistry of detoxification, around 80 per cent of all the building that the body does is for the purposes of detoxification. The end-products of Phase 1 are transformed by 'sticking' things on to them in a process called conjugation. Some toxins have glutathione stuck to them (glutathione conjugation). This is how we detoxify paracetamol (acetaminophen), for example. In cases of overdose, a person is given glutathione to mop up the highly destructive toxins generated by Phase 1 detoxification of this drug.

Other toxins have sulphur stuck to them in a process called sulphation. This is the fate of many steroid hormones, neurotransmitters and, once again, paracetamol. The sulphur comes directly from food. Garlic, onions and eggs are good sources of sulphur-containing amino acids such as methionine and cysteine – so if you lack these you've got a problem. Others have carbon compounds, called methyl groups, stuck to them (this is called methylation). Lead and arsenic are detoxified in this way. Aspirin has the amino acid glycine stuck to it (this is called glycine conjugation). When these pathways are overloaded, the body can use another, known as glucuronidation, which is the primary route for breaking down many tranquillisers.

TOO MANY TOXINS OR NOT ENOUGH NUTRIENTS?

When these biochemical pathways don't work properly, due to overload or a lack of nutrients, the body generates harmful toxins. An example is homocysteine, a toxic byproduct of breaking down the amino acid methionine. This can be a result of problems with sulphation (usually due to a lack of vitamin B6) or methylation (which involves folic acid and B12). Sulphur dioxide, a component of exhaust fumes, is detoxified via the sulphation pathway whose enzymes depend on the mineral molybdenum, which is particularly high in beans. Over-exposure, coupled with a molybdenum-deficient diet, can lead to intolerance of exhaust fumes.

These detoxifying pathways work together. If one is overloaded, a toxin may be processed by another. Homocysteine can, as a back-up, be mopped up by glycine conjugation, which is why taking in more of the amino acid glycine often has the effect of lowering an elevated homocysteine level.

LIVER PROBLEMS OR HEALTH PROBLEMS?

Taking a liver's eye view of disease processes often sheds new light on some common health problems of the late twentieth century. For example, just about any allergic, inflammatory or metabolic disorder, including eczema, asthma, chronic fatigue, chronic infections, inflammatory bowel disorders, multiple sclerosis, rheumatoid arthritis, and even schizophrenia and hormone imbalances, may involve or create sub-optimum liver function.

Many hormone-related problems are currently blamed on 'oestrogen dominance'. The body makes oestrogen and maintains the right balance by a series of processes in the liver. The balance of oestrone, oestradiol and oestriol (the three oestrogenic hormones) is critical to health. The transformation of one into another and their degradation is controlled by the liver. So poor liver function can lead to an imbalance and accumulation of oestrogenic hormones.

The brain is not able to disarm a wide range of toxins – it

depends on the liver to do a chemical clean-up of the blood before it gets there. So toxic overload of the liver has dire consequences for brain and nervous system function. Autism, schizophrenia and memory loss are all associated with poor liver function. A classic example is alcoholism. When the liver can't deal with the quantity of alcohol consumed, the brain is left unprotected. This is why brain damage, dementia and mental illness are some particularly unpleasant consequences of chronic alcohol abuse.

CHOLESTEROL AND BLOOD SUGAR CONTROL

Cholesterol is both made and detoxified by the liver. If you need more, it will make it. If you need less, it will break it down – if it can. Cholesterol is a major building block for hormones. Your body can use it to make the sex hormones testosterone, oestrogen and progesterone as well as adrenal hormones. From cholesterol, the liver can make bile to digest fat. The body makes no less than 1 litre of bile each day. Although most is re-absorbed from the digestive tract into the blood, the small amount that leaves the body takes with it toxins excreted by the liver. Liver problems usually lead to an accumulation of fat in the liver which can be responsible for 'fatty liver' or 'sluggish liver', associated with excess alcohol consumption.

The liver can also turn sugar into glycogen and fat. When your blood sugar level is low it turns glycogen back into glucose. By ensuring optimal liver function, you improve your body's ability to maintain the right balance of cholesterol, triglycerides (blood fats) and glucose, which are vital to maintaining good health.

TESTING LIVER FUNCTION

Standard tests for liver function involve measuring levels of the key enzymes GPT (glutamate-pyruvate transaminase) and GOT (glutamate-oxaloacetate transaminase). If they are raised, it means your liver is struggling. This is an indication of a chronic problem and, while it is useful in pinpointing that a problem exists, it doesn't really identify the best way to help recovery.

A more advanced and detailed indication of liver function, capable of picking up imbalances before they develop into chronic health problems, is a Comprehensive Detoxification Profile. This is a non-invasive test that involves ingesting a measured amount of caffeine, aspirin and paracetamol and then analysing certain chemicals that appear in the urine. How these substances are dealt with and what they turn into helps determine which pathways are working and which ones aren't. If one pathway is under-functioning, another may be over-functioning to help cope with the load.

Some people with toxic overload – perhaps from over-exposure to exo-toxins, or a gut infection in which the disease-causing organism generates toxins, or a leaky gut in which toxic substances are more easily able to enter the body – become 'pathological detoxifiers'. This means their Phase 1 system is hyperactive, trying to get the endless rubbish ready for collection. Phase 2 processes, meanwhile, are overloaded and simply can't deal with all the toxins being generated. In these cases, just giving a person a lot of B vitamins could make them worse, not better, because these nutrients further speed up Phase 1, thus increasing the overload on the Phase 2 processes.

RESTORING OPTIMAL LIVER FUNCTION

The good news is that, with a good diet, lifestyle and the right supplements, you can restore and maintain optimal liver function. For people with long-term health problems, especially those involving chronic fatigue, allergies, chemical sensitivities or digestive disorders, it is well worth seeing a clinical nutritionist and having the necessary tests. They can help to identify the sources of toxic overload and how to eliminate them, and recommend the right balance of nutrients to get the liver's log-jam moving again. For personal guidance and referral for a Comprehensive Detoxification Profile, you should consult a clinical nutritionist (see Useful Addresses).

Prevention, however, is better than cure, so if you are basically healthy and want to promote and maintain optimal liver function the best advice is to cut down on your intake of toxic substances, eat an optimal diet and take a balanced nutrition supplement programme. In practice, this means you should:

- Minimise your intake of alcohol, caffeine, cigarettes, sugar, fried foods, saturated fat, pesticides, exhaust fumes and medications.
- Increase your intake of all fruits and vegetables, especially those rich in antioxidants (carrots, tomatoes, green peppers, watercress, etc); anthocyanidins (berries, beetroot, grapes); and glucosinolates (cabbage, broccoli, Brussels sprouts, kale). Eat carnivorous fish in place of meat, and cold-pressed seeds and seed oils instead of butter; and drink plenty of purified water. Artichokes and turmeric also aid liver function.
- Supplement a high-strength multivitamin and mineral, additional antioxidant nutrients and at least 2000mg of vitamin C. Some supplement companies also produce specific nutrient combinations designed to support liver function. Nutrients that can specifically help the liver are choline, methionine, liver extract and the herbs milk thistle (contains silymarin) and dandelion root.

CHAPTER 18

SOLVING THE RIDDLE OF IRRITABLE BOWEL SYNDROME

Irritable Bowel Syndrome (IBS) does not paint a clear picture. Rather, it appears to be a broad term used to describe several, sometimes contradictory symptoms. The effects can be random and can disappear as spontaneously as they come on, although for many people it is a chronic condition. All this apparent vagueness does not make for an easy diagnosis or treatment but, with such a high incidence, this problem – also known as intestinal neurosis, spastic colitis, spastic colon, mucous colitis – demands a solution. Many sufferers find anti-spasmodic drugs, fibre supplements and laxatives prescribed by their doctors unhelpful. IBS is the second highest cause of absenteeism after the common cold, with 20 per cent of the adult population experiencing bouts of it. Twice as many women as men are said to suffer from it, although this may just be because women are more likely to report the symptoms.

If you have any or all the following symptoms, continually or recurrently for at least three months, there is a strong possibility that you have IBS:

Symptoms of IBS

- abdominal pain
- anxiety
- bloating
- constipation
- cramps
- depression
- diarrhoea
- gas
- mucus in stools
- nausea

Whatever the cause of the symptoms that can be described as IBS, the common thread is a disturbance to the usual control of the bowel by a complex set of nerves which determines its movements and the substances it secretes. Normally, digestion is regulated in part by the autonomic branch of the nervous system (ANS), which controls involuntary bodily functions such as the beating of the heart and the secretion of hormones. In a healthy gut, the ANS moves food along with rhythmic contractions, but in the case of IBS the muscles go into spasm. The mechanisms by which the ANS works are very subtle and therefore easily disrupted. When this happens, food and waste material does not move along the digestive tract normally, so mucus and toxins accumulate; gas and stools become trapped, causing bloating and pain, which often worsens with eating and is relieved by a bowel movement. Women often find their symptoms worsen around the time of their period.

IBS OR INFLAMMATORY BOWEL DISEASE?

One distinguishing feature of IBS – compared with other bowel complaints – is that there are no particular changes visible in bowel tissue (as with Crohn's disease, in which the digestive tract becomes ulcerated). Another feature of IBS sufferers is that, despite symptoms, their overall health is good, without the serious factors such as weight loss, fever, bleeding or anaemia that come with other bowel disorders. Before any treatment of suspected IBS, it is important to get a GP to rule out other conditions that may be linked to similar symptoms: diverticulitis, infectious diarrhoea, inflammatory bowel disease (e.g. Crohn's or ulcerative colitis), diabetes, cancer, laxative abuse, mechanical problems such as impacted faeces, coeliac disease and others.

Back in 1892, Sir William Osler, in *The Principles and Practice of Medicine*, wrote of mucous colitis, describing 'a tenacious mucus, which may be slimy and gelatinous, like frog-spawn' in patients who were often hysterical and depressed. So IBS is not entirely a modern disease, yet the alarming prevalence of IBS in developed countries is just one indication that it is a condition which is largely due to diet and lifestyle. There is no quick fix though. 'Unfortunately, there's no single cause for IBS, but hopefully we can find the causes for each person and work with them individually in response to their biochemical uniqueness,' explains Elizabeth Lipski in *Digestive Wellness*.

Because there is no test for IBS as such, it is essential to create a picture of what is causing the symptoms for each individual – be it food allergies, stress, hormone changes, dietary factors including low fibre, infection or other factors. A practitioner therefore has to take a careful history of the client's symptoms, diet and lifestyle in order to determine the cause of the IBS. Dr Jean Munro, Medical Director of the Brakespear Hospital for Allergy and Environmental Medicine, believes, 'It's practically always associated with food reactions as well as some form of dysbiosis.'

IBS AND ALLERGIES

Food sensitivities in people with IBS have been recognised since the turn of the century and are found in as many as two-thirds of sufferers. In people who have allergies or come from families with allergies, this must be a prime consideration. Clinical studies have found the most commonly offending foods to be grains (especially wheat), dairy products, coffee, tea and citrus fruits. Intolerance of lactose (the sugar in milk) is particularly common; while other sugars, even those in fruits, can cause problems too. Many IBS sufferers find relief by avoiding gluten (wheat, oats, rye, barley), but it is usually those with diarrhoea who find they do better without dairy products. The most suitable test for food sensitivities is the ELISA IgE/IgG test, although it is usually more conclusive (and considerably cheaper) to use an elimination diet (see Chapter 11).

Food intolerances are frequently linked to leaky gut syndrome (see Chapter 16). This in itself can cause a host of problems, including depressed immunity and fatigue. If IBS is persistent, it may well be linked to leaky gut, in which case steps must be taken to heal the gut lining using dietary changes and supplements such as zinc, vitamin A, essential fatty acids, glutamine and N-acetyl-glucosamine. Tests are available to determine gut permeability.

Other problems of digestion are also linked to IBS: a lack of digestive enzymes due to genetic factors, age, smoking, etc will mean that food is not broken down properly, causing fermentation, leaky gut and other conditions which cause or exacerbate IBS. Some foods, such as pulses, beans, nuts and cauliflower, contain a carbohydrate that is inherently difficult to digest. A special digestive enzyme – alpha-galactosidase – helps break it down.

Other than intolerances of specific foods, a diet low in nutrients, fresh foods and fibre (not wheat bran, which can irritate the gut) can trigger digestive and other disorders. It invariably causes constipation and an imbalance in gut flora (dysbiosis) which ultimately causes a build-up of toxic matter in the lining of the intestines; IBS is just one possible outcome. During an attack of IBS, it's best to have bland, easily digestible foods, fresh juices (especially carrot and apple), slippery elm tea and other soothing drinks. Charcoal tablets can be used to relieve occasional gas and bloating; but it is important to eliminate the cause, rather than just dealing with the symptoms.

Use the following list of general dietary tips to help alleviate IBS:

- Eliminate suspected allergenic foods.
- Eat plenty of fresh vegetables.
- Eat simple meals and chew thoroughly.
- Increase dietary fibre (not wheat bran), especially in cases of constipation.
- Drink plenty of water, herbal teas and diluted juices.
- Avoid foods rich in sulphur as they can cause wind (bread, eggs, onions and most dried fruits).
- Avoid sugar.
- Avoid wheat (even in people who are not sensitive, it can irritate the gut).
- Avoid refined/processed foods.
- Avoid animal fats and dairy products (especially in cases of diarrhoea).
- Limit or avoid alcohol, coffee, tea and cigarettes.
- Avoid spicy foods.

As we have seen, we all have numerous bacteria and other micro-organisms living in our guts. Problems arise when 'unfriendly' bacteria outnumber the good ones, or are toxic, or others (such as yeasts) multiply to such an extent that they disrupt digestive function. Such imbalances (discussed fully in

Chapters 13 and 15) often accompany IBS. Using antibiotics and antacids can contribute to dysbiosis by disturbing the delicate balance of microflora throughout the digestive tract. Altering your diet and taking supplements of beneficial bacteria (or other substances, such as butyric acid or fructo-oligosaccharides, that encourage their growth) will help to repopulate the intestinal environment with these essential friends. An overgrowth of the yeast *Candida albicans*, a relatively common problem which sometimes accompanies IBS, requires special dietary strategies (discussed in Chapter 15).

The number of parasites that inhabit our intestines may be quite alarming; most produce no symptoms, but others can give rise to IBS, gastro-intestinal disorders and other health problems (see Chapter 14).

THE STRESS CONNECTION

As mentioned, the functioning of the digestive tract is subject to the intricate workings of the autonomic nervous system (ANS) which we do not consciously control, and any disruption to this can have far-reaching effects. Stress to the body – whether it is a strong emotion, anxiety, illness, or even the presence of an allergenic food or toxin – will set alarm bells ringing. In such a situation, the ANS perceives 'danger' and diverts energy from systems – such as digestion – that are not immediately required to deal with the 'emergency'. As you can imagine, shutting down the digestive system is likely to result in constipation and a build-up of toxins. In some situations the ANS reaction is so strong that it results in immediate diarrhoea.

Obviously, not everyone who gets stressed (i.e. all of us, at some time) suffers from IBS, but there is a clear link between the two. An article in *The Lancet* suggests that 'anxiety is a predisposing factor'. The other side of the coin is that people suffering from a long-term, frustrating condition such as IBS are likely to become anxious or depressed, as shown in numerous studies. Whichever comes first – IBS or stress of any sort – many sufferers have found great relief when they combine treatment with behavioural therapies such as stress management, counselling or hypnotherapy. Herbs such as skullcap, valerian and passionflower can be useful for calming the ANS. Other practices – such as yoga, T'ai Chi, regular exercise, taking time to eat, chewing well and not eating less than two hours before bedtime – also promote better digestive function.

With so many possible triggers of IBS, care needs to be taken in formulating a treatment programme. It is important to investigate the underlying factors for each individual and deal with these, rather than simply treating the symptoms. A majority of IBS sufferers find that increasing dietary fibre helps enormously, especially for those with constipation. Fibre not only helps make bowel movements more regular in the short term, but also tones intestinal muscles, keeps the gut lining 'cleaner', and helps balance gut flora. However, the type of fibre used is important. Wheat bran, a popular choice, can sometimes do more harm than good, not just because wheat itself is a common allergen but also because the bran actually irritates the intestinal lining. Fruit and vegetable fibre, on the other hand, as well as other grains (such as brown rice, rye and quinoa) can benefit many people with IBS. People with diarrhoea must be careful, as some fibre may aggravate them – pectin (apples, bananas) and algin (seaweeds) may be helpful. If you increase the fibre in your diet it is important also to drink more water.

Alongside a wholefood diet free from refined foods, there are several supplements – vitamins, minerals, essential fats, amino acids, herbs and other botanical preparations – which can help immensely. Supporting the liver with these is also an important part of the cleansing and healing process (see Chapter 17). Vitamin B complex, for example, is needed for proper muscle tone, for the absorption of foods, for repair, for metabolising foods and generally in our response to stress. Magnesium can help reduce muscle spasms; alfalfa helps promote healthy intestinal flora, healing and cleansing; and peppermint oil (enterically coated to make sure it is not absorbed in the stomach) is widely used to relieve the symptoms of IBS.

A clinical nutritionist (see Useful Addresses) can help you identify which supplements will best suit your individual needs, and advise on lifestyle practices that can help alleviate IBS. The symptoms of irritable bowel syndrome can be overcome by diet, supplements, exercise and relaxation; although the process may take a while, it can ultimately allow most people who have it to lead fulfilling, active lives.

CHAPTER 19

CONQUERING CROHN'S, COLITIS AND DIVERTICULITIS

Unlike the broader and more nebulous 'diagnosis' of irritable bowel syndrome, Crohn's, colitis and diverticulitis are all inflammatory diseases that can actually be diagnosed by the presence of inflammation along the digestive tract. While the advice for irritable bowel syndrome holds true in these cases too, the emphasis in correcting these conditions should be on removing the causes of inflammation, reducing the inflammation itself and healing the digestive tract.

Diverticula are pockets which form in the large intestine that can become inflamed – causing diverticulitis – primarily as a consequence of eating a poor, low-fibre diet. This can also be true for milder cases of colitis (inflammation of the colon), which is quite different from Crohn's and ulcerative colitis. These are the two major types of what is known as inflammatory bowel disease, or IBD for short. They are much more complex, involving abnormal immune system responses, possibly allergies, intestinal permeability and genetic factors. Crohn's and ulcerative colitis now affect one in every 1000 people and, without proper treatment, can necessitate surgery to remove the damaged section of the digestive tract.

Whether a person is diagnosed with Crohn's or ulcerative colitis depends on the location and type of inflammation, as well as the symptoms. Ulcerative colitis causes inflammation of the lining of the colon only; classic symptoms are passing blood and mucus, pain before defecation, a general feeling of tiredness and, in more severe cases, diarrhoea. Crohn's disease can affect any part of the bowel, usually the last part of the small intestine (the ileum), in a more severe way, thickening the intestinal wall, often with normal bowel in between inflamed sections.

INFLAMMATORY BOWEL DISEASE – A COMPLEX EQUATION

While there is no one universal therapy for inflammatory bowel disease, a complex picture is emerging of a number of causative factors which together lead to inflammation of the bowel. These factors include:

- genetically inherited tendency towards inflammation
- certain food allergies or sensitivities
- dysbiosis, including bacterial imbalance and infections
- increased intestinal permeability
- detoxification problems.

In a study of children in the Newcastle district, researchers from the Royal Victoria Infirmary found that those with Crohn's disease had a sixfold increase in intestinal permeability.[13] In another study at St Bartholomew's Hospital in London, children with Crohn's disease and intestinal permeability were fed a diet of pure nutrients (not food as such) for six weeks. As a consequence there was both a substantial improvement in their symptoms and in their intestinal permeability.[14] Indeed, many researchers have found that low-allergenic diets can produce significant relief both from Crohn's and ulcerative colitis. The most common offending foods are wheat, milk and yeast, although the ideal diet varies from person to person.

The first step in its correction is therefore to identify the offending foods and eliminate them. The next step is to correct dysbiosis and re-inoculate the digestive tract with the right beneficial bacteria. There is some evidence that the wrong balance of bacteria may generate toxins that then damage the intestinal wall. The wrong bacterial imbalance can also affect immune function, leading to increased inflammation in the digestive tract, so balancing this is important. The amino acid glutamine is especially important in healing the digestive tract.

The main medical treatment is the use of anti-inflammatory drugs to calm down the inflammation, or medication to turn off the body's immune reactions. These drugs are effective but do nothing to address the actual causes of the inflammation. According to Dr Jeffrey Bland, a pioneer in new approaches to inflammation, 'Instead of thinking "pain means drug", inflammation is the body's way of saying something is wrong. Inflammation is a "systemic" problem, not just a localised phenomenon, in which the body's physiology is shifted into an "alarm" state.' It's as if there is a series of underlying imbalances in the body's chemistry that build up and then burst forth, when the body can no longer cope with a set of circumstances. The actual pain is the wave breaking, although the wave is a long time coming.

From this perspective, there are several factors that set the scene for inflammation, and then those which trigger the manifestation of symptoms. So often it's the 'hair that broke the camel's back' that gets the blame. 'My colitis started when

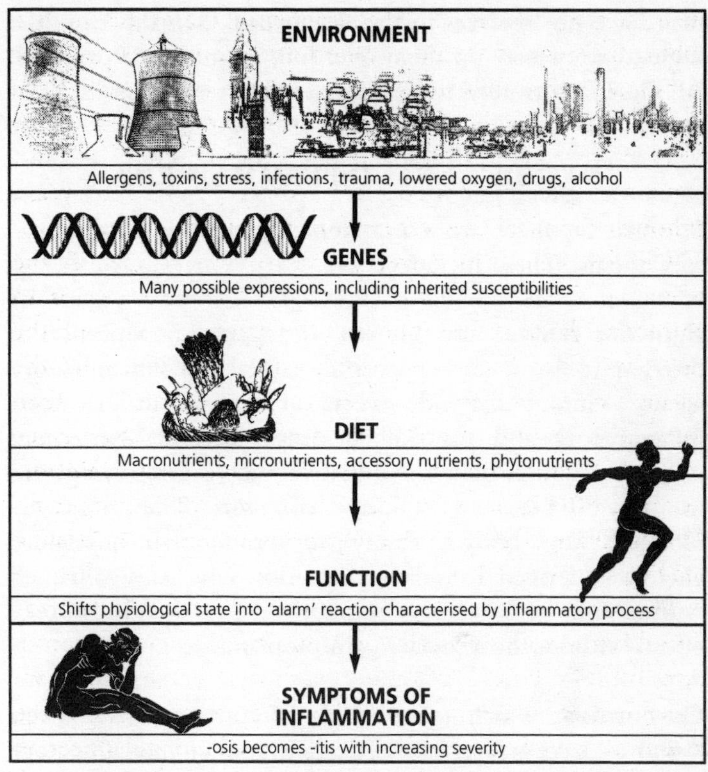

Figure 15 – The inflammatory process

my marriage was breaking up' or 'Ever since I had that bout of flu I started to get abdominal pain'. These triggers are important and may include a trauma, an allergy, an infection, a toxin or exposure to too many oxidants. Indeed, recent research has indicated that the triple vaccine for measles, mumps and rubella (MMR), which effectively induces all of these infections, increases the risk of developing Crohn's. One would hope that a healthy person could rise to such challenges, but if there are underlying weaknesses, such as a genetic predisposition or poor nutritional status, the person may have no 'reserves in the health bank'. In this case, the slightest stress may tip them over into an inflammatory state. All these factors need to be considered to restore health.

NATURE'S ANTI-INFLAMMATORIES

Fortunately, there are a number of natural anti-inflammatory agents. These include:

Boswellia serrata, also known as Indian Frankincense, is proving to be a very powerful natural anti-inflammatory agent, without the side-effects of current drugs. Anti-inflammatory and pain-killing drugs such as aspirin and phenylbutazone irritate the digestive tract, causing symptoms in over 20 per cent of long-term users. They work by blocking the body's ability to produce inflammatory chemicals, derived from dietary fats. Boswellic acids contained within the herb achieve comparative anti-inflammatory effects without the associated gut problems.

Curcumins, which are extracts of turmeric, have been found to have powerful antioxidant and anti-inflammatory properties. Curcumins have a similar mode of action to boswellic acid and, together with a good optimum nutrition programme including anti-inflammatory essential fats, may prove at least as effective as drugs.

Fish oils high in omega 3 fats, particularly EPA and DHA, are well established in fighting inflammation. These natural, anti-inflammatory fats are particularly abundant in fish with teeth, which eat fish that eat plankton. Each step up the food chain concentrates them.

This natural approach to conquering inflammatory bowel disease is complex, like the problem itself, and is best effected by working with a qualified clinical nutritionist (see Useful Addresses). A nutritionist can run the necessary tests and advise you on diet and supplements for each stage of eliminating the cause of the inflammation, calming it and helping to repair the damaged gut. This approach is based on an understanding that inflammation and pain are the body's way of saying 'help' and that current diet and lifestyle factors have exceeded the body's capacity to adapt. Rather than suppressing the inflammation with drugs, it aims to identify the contributing factors and restore balance.

CHAPTER 20

Preventing Wind, Bloating, Constipation and Haemorrhoids

The digestive tract usually contains about 200ml of gas, and it is not abnormal to pass 400–2000ml of this daily. About 90 per cent of the gas is made up of nitrogen, oxygen, carbon dioxide, methane and hydrogen. The nitrogen and oxygen come from air that is swallowed; the carbon dioxide is produced when stomach acid mixes with bicarbonates in bile and pancreatic juices. Most of the oxygen and carbon dioxide are reabsorbed into the bloodstream through the small intestine. The colon, or large bowel, contains billions of bacteria, which are essential for good health (see Chapter 13) and whose job it is to ferment products which pass from the small intestine. As the bacteria ferment the residues, large amounts of hydrogen, methane, carbon dioxide and other gases are produced. Although some of these are reabsorbed into the blood and excreted in the breath, the rest is passed as wind.

THE CAUSES OF WIND

One of the major causes of excessive wind is indigestion. If food is not completely broken down this provides micro-organisms in the digestive tract with more 'food' – hence more gas. So the first step to solving this problem is to change your diet and supplement digestive enzymes with each meal (see Chapter 3). Certain foods do generate more gas, including beans and certain vegetables such as cabbage, Brussels sprouts, cauliflower, turnips, leeks, onions and garlic. A high-fibre diet is also likely to generate more gas. This is because these foods contain indigestible carbohydrates. One of the main types of indigestible carbohydrates are galactosides. While a small amount of gas from eating these foods is quite normal, excessive gas can be prevented by supplementing the enzyme alpha-galactosidase. This breaks down these indigestible carbohydrates and reduces flatulence. Some digestive enzyme formulas contain this enzyme as well as enzymes that digest protein, fat and carbohydrate. Excessive and foul-smelling wind is usually eliminated by changing your diet and following the steps in Part 4 to restore digestive health.

Another cause of wind is dysbiosis. An infection with *Candida albicans*, for example, or an excess of the 'bad' gut bacteria can all contribute to excessive wind. People taking antibiotics, which disturb the healthy balance of bacteria, often find they pass more wind. Correcting bacterial imbalance with probiotics (see Chapter 13) often reduces this problem, although it can make matters worse in the first week as the beneficial bacteria re-establish themselves.

If too much air gets into the stomach – from eating quickly, gulping food, drinking too much liquid with food, chewing gum, smoking or drinking fizzy drinks which generate carbon dioxide – it is relieved by belching. This is perfectly normal. Sometimes, as part of a stress reaction, people take in too much air. The effects of stress on digestion are discussed in the next chapter.

BLOATING

Bloating and abdominal distention are usually the result of the same factors that cause flatulence. Excessive bloating, especially if the abdominal area becomes very distended and hard like a full balloon, contributes to intestinal permeability (see Chapter 16) and is therefore a sign of an unhealthy digestive system. Bloating can also be due to irregularities in which the muscles don't work properly to keep everything moving along, often resulting in constipation or, at least, sluggish digestion.

CONSTIPATION

Constipation has many causes, the most common of which is hard faecal matter. Natural foods stay soft in the digestive tract because they contain fibres which absorb water and expand inside the digestive tract. Fruits and vegetables naturally contain a lot of water in themselves. Provided they are prepared properly, whole grains, such as oats and rice, absorb water and provide watery bulk for the digestive tract. Given that we are literally 65 per cent water, it makes sense to eat foods with a high water content. Meats, cheese, eggs, refined grains and wheat (because of its gluten content) can all be constipating. While it should not be necessary to add fibre to a good diet, oat fibre has particular benefits. This is naturally present in oats which are best soaked and eaten cold. Some foods and nutrients exert a mild laxative effect, such as linseed (which can be ground and sprinkled on food), prunes and also vitamin C (in doses of several grams).

Not drinking enough water is a major cause of constipation. We need at least 1 litre of water a day for optimal digestive health and this alone often relieves constipation.

With the right high-fibre diet and enough water, a person should experience the need to defecate two or three times a day, after meals. Stools should be loosely formed, rather than hard. Many people suppress or ignore the natural need to go to the toilet, which, in itself, generates constipation. So, if you have the slightest urge to defecate after a meal, go for it. Disturbances in the normal peristaltic muscle action of the bowel can also lead to constipation and a suppression of this natural reflex. This is discussed in the next chapter.

Natural laxatives

Most laxatives, even natural laxatives containing the herbs senna or cascara, are gastro-intestinal irritants and, although they work, they don't really solve the underlying issue. They may be useful as an emergency measure, but it is not a good idea to be taking such remedies on a continual basis. Some remedies aimed at promoting regularity are concentrated fibre preparations containing things like bran, ispaghula, methylcellulose or sterculia. It is very important to drink plenty of water if you are taking such fibre supplements. However, as you start to change towards a high-fibre diet, they should not be necessary.

A new kind of laxative, fructo-oligosaccharides (FOS), provided as a powder, work in a more beneficial way than conventional laxatives, which can make it harder to re-establish proper peristaltic muscle action. FOS are a type of complex carbohydrate that helps keep moisture in the gut and also stimulates production of healthy bacteria. This keeps faecal matter softer and easier to pass along. While results are not quite so rapid, this is a highly preferable way of reducing constipation.

The consequences of constipation

For some people long-term constipation can result in physical blockages and distentions of the bowel. This is the major cause of diverticulosis and can lead to inflammatory bowel problems (see Chapter 19). Constipation slows down the time food spends in the digestive tract, which allows more opportunity for putrefaction and exposure to toxic material. This is a major contributor to colo-rectal cancer and it is therefore no surprise to find that there is an association between constipation and increased risk of colo-rectal cancer.[15]

Haemorrhoids (Piles)

Another consequence of chronic constipation is haemorrhoids. These are swollen blood vessels in and around the anus and rectum that stretch under pressure, much like a varicose vein. The most common reason for the development of haemorrhoids is straining on defecation. Therefore, the less compacted and softer the stool, the easier it is to pass. The main symptom of haemorrhoids is anal itching (which can be present in candidiasis infection or in inflammatory bowel disease), which, in turn, can lead to excessive scratching, which further aggravates the condition. Diarrhoea can also aggravate anal itching and hence stress can aggravate haemorrhoids. While frequent warm baths and anti-inflammatory creams can relieve symptoms, long-term relief is achieved, as for constipation, by dietary changes.

Dietary changes help but are not always enough to completely cleanse the intestinal tract. A combination of particular fibres, such as psyllium husks, beet fibre, oat fibre and herbs, which help loosen up old faecal material, can be beneficial. These are available in colon-cleansing formulas, consisting of powders and capsules to be taken over a one-to three-month period (see Chapter 24).

Another helpful treatment is colonic therapy. This is an advanced enema where water is passed into the bowel and, together with abdominal massage, helps to release and remove old faecal material.

Exercise that stimulates the abdominal area can also improve digestion, as do breathing exercises that relax the abdomen. It is a natural reflex of the body to stop digesting in times of stress, so relaxation is important, as you will see in the next chapter.

CHAPTER 21

STRESS, ABDOMINAL TENSION AND PERISTALSIS

The digestive system cannot be separated from the rest of the body, nor the body from the mind. Our level of stress and psychological state therefore have a lot to do with digestive health. The digestive system is the basis of our survival, so it represents the instinct for self-preservation. Its physical territory is the abdominal cavity and its centre is the belly. In the martial arts tradition the centre of vital energy is located in a point four fingerwidths below the belly-button and about 2.5cm in. This is known in different traditions as the *kath*, *ki* or *tan-tien*.

The abdominal cavity is separated from the thoracic cavity (lungs, heart and kidneys, contained within the rib cage) by the diaphragm, a dome-shaped muscle. The way we breathe and the action of the diaphragm muscle are critical to our digestive processes. In a relaxed and healthy person the diaphragm muscle is pulled downwards as we inhale, opening up lung space for air to enter; and it is contracted upwards, reducing lung space as we exhale. Therefore the belly should extend as we inhale, as the diaphragm muscle descends, and it should relax on the out-breath. This is what happens in babies

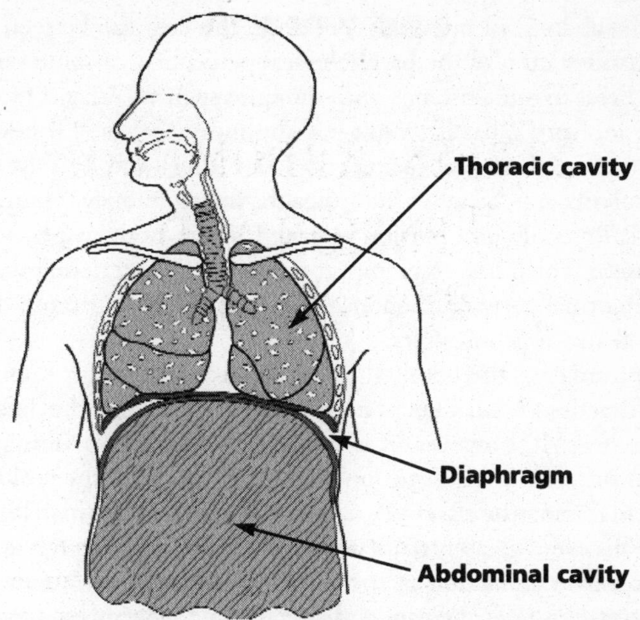

Figure 16 – The abdominal and thoracic cavity and the diaphragm muscle

and in animals but, as we get older, many of us lose this natural, deep breathing ability and instead take very shallow breaths. It is almost as if these two cavities have become disconnected which, in turn, means the digestive organs do not get 'massaged' by the movements of the diaphragm muscle. It also means the muscles of the abdomen may stay in a state of tension, inhibiting the digestive processes.

While the heart, or thoracic cavity, is said to represent our instinct to relate to others, the belly or abdominal cavity is connected to our instinct for self-preservation, our 'being'. The head or cranial cavity represents our adaptation instinct, our 'doing'. Psychological tensions about doing (coping), relating (belonging) and being (feeling safe) manifest in the body as physical tension. One major area of physical tension is the abdominal muscles. Tension in this area can be seen as a manifestation of the psychological perception of some kind of threat to our existence with thoughts such as 'What if I lose my job' or 'What if I can't pay the mortgage' or 'I'll never have enough to feel secure' or 'I don't feel safe' (i.e. issues involving our being – food, health, home, money, security etc). Psychological tension is stored in the body as physical tension which has a real impact on digestion, interfering with the normal peristaltic action of the muscles that surround the small and large intestines.

Normally, this peristaltic, snake-like wave of muscle contractions is what keeps everything moving along the digestive tract. If, however, it is suppressed, either by abdominal tension or by constipation and distention of the colon, peristalsis may be effectively blocked or weakened, which leads to an even greater tendency to constipation. Conversely, excessive contraction of the abdominal muscles can result in cramp-like digestive pain and a tendency to diarrhoea.

RELAXING THE BELLY AND RE-ESTABLISHING PERISTALSIS

There are several ways to restore proper abdominal muscle tone and peristalsis. These include methods of breathing, abdominal exercises, massage, colonic therapy and muscle-relaxing herbs. All these approaches can be helpful for a wide variety of digestive problems, from abdominal cramping and irritable bowel syndrome (see Chapter 18), to constipation and indigestion. So too can tackling the psychological issues and stresses that lead to abdominal tension.

Breathing exercises

Different schools of yoga and martial arts teach various breathing exercises designed to encourage full, deep breathing, which strengthens and fully utilises the diaphragm muscle. One method I particularly like is called *dia-kath* breathing and is part of an exercise system known as Psychocalisthenics. In essence, the exercise involves imagining the *kath* point as a magnet which attracts the diaphragm muscle downwards on inhaling. This visualisation, under proper instruction, soon generates very much deeper breathing from the belly. This not only improves digestive health but also substantially improves oxygen supply and exchange, in turn generating increased vitality.

Abdominal exercises

Conventional exercise focuses on 'pulling in the belly' to look slim and, in men, developing the 'six-pack' look, but it is also important for the abdominal area to be able to

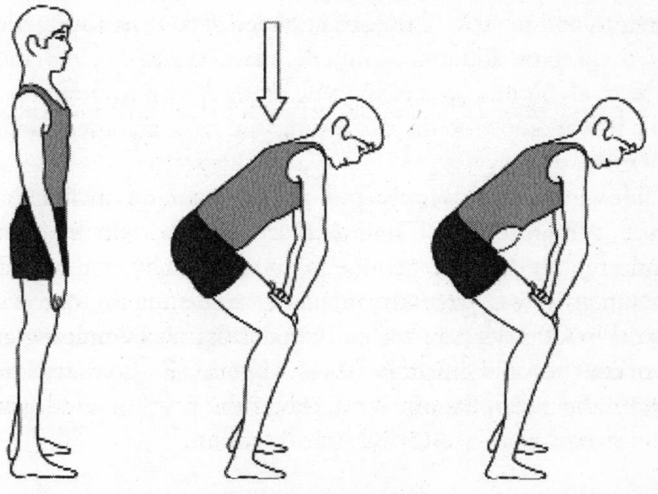

Foot Position: 3 foot-widths
Breathing: *Inhale*, 3 beats *Exhale*, 3 beats
Hold breath, contract and release muscles, 9 beats
Repeat 3 times.

Figure 17 – Udiyama

relax properly and extend with the breath. So, while abdominal muscle-strengthening exercises such as sit-ups are good, you also need other kinds of abdominal exercise such as Udiyama, a classic yoga exercise that helps stimulate digestion and massages the organs in the abdominal region.

Bend your knees and place your hands on your thighs just above the knees with your fingers pointing inward. Your shoulders, arms and hands are relaxed. Your spine and neck are straight. To get the correct 45 degree inclination, bend your knees and tilt your torso and head forward, bringing your hands to rest lightly on your thighs. Your head and spine are in a straight line. Avoid bending over too far. Check the buttock muscles; they should remain relaxed. Exhale sharply, empty your lungs and force the stomach out. Keeping the lungs empty, alternately contract and relax the abdominal muscles in rapid succession nine times. Make each contraction as deep as possible. Keep the movements of the belly smooth and regular. The correct stance makes the contraction of the rectus abdominis muscle massage the viscera most effectively. You can feel the pull from the pubis bone up to the throat. Do not do this exercise if you are pregnant or menstruating.

However, this is only one of 23 exercises included in the 20-minute Psychocalisthenics routine, which, in its entirety, represents a wonderful way to enliven the body, maintain fitness, strength, suppleness and improve digestion (see Useful Addresses for further details). A complete yoga workout would include such abdominal exercises plus others for rejuvenation.

Massage

Although conventional massage rarely delves into releasing tension in the abdominal region, a good massage therapist can encourage the release of abdominal tension. Most of us hold tension in that area, especially when we are under stress. However, care must be taken with such massage in people with inflammatory bowel disease.

Colonic therapy

During a 'colonic', water is passed gently into the colon and this stimulates the peristaltic muscle action. A good colonic therapist (see Useful Addresses) massages the abdominal area during the session in a way that encourages peristaltic muscle action. To re-establish peristaltic muscle action, which can be felt much like a heartbeat, it is best to see a colonic therapist every two or three days until peristalsis is back to normal. This is very helpful for people with a history of constipation, although it would be best to start it after a couple of months of good dietary practices.

Muscle-relaxing herbs

Peppermint is a powerful muscle-relaxing herb. Peppermint oil capsules have proven highly effective in people who have abdominal muscle cramping, particularly in irritable bowel syndrome. These capsules are swallowed, then released in the stomach and upper part of the digestive tract and, if muscle contraction is part of the problem, can provide significant and relatively immediate relief. However, bear in mind that such muscle contractions can often be the body's way of saying that it is not receiving what it needs in terms of healing foods. So look closely at what you are eating.

CHAPTER 22

SAY NO TO DIGESTIVE CANCERS

Cancers of the digestive tract are, more often than not, the consequence of long-term insult due to poor diet, infections and digestive irritants. Cancers of the digestive tract itself (mouth, oesophagus, stomach, colon and rectum) are most strongly linked to diet, while cancer of the liver and pancreas are somewhat more nebulous in origin. In any event, following the advice for restoring digestive health in Part 4 of this book is the best way to minimise your risk.

MOUTH, THROAT AND OESOPHAGUS CANCER

The location of these cancers is strongly suggestive of ingested or inhaled carcinogens. Known risk factors are alcohol, smoking, lack of fruit and vegetables, high intake of maté tea or very hot drinks. The combination of smoking and drinking particularly increases the risk of oesophageal cancer. The most protective nutrients are antioxidants, especially vitamin C, vitamin A and selenium, alongside a diet high in fruit and vegetables and low in alcohol. Don't have very hot drinks and, needless to say, avoid smoking.

STOMACH CANCER

Stomach cancer affects 12 000 people a year in the UK. It is very strongly linked to dietary carcinogens, so it is prevented both by avoiding high-risk foods and having a good intake of nutrients which can disarm carcinogens in food. Known contributory factors are: an excess of salt and salted foods; grilled, fried, barbecued or burnt meat; a lack of refrigeration which increases the risk of pathogens in food; low intake of fresh fruit and vegetables.

Stomach cancer starts in the lining of the stomach – which is normally protected from damage by mucus secretions – so it is very likely that digestive irritation is a key trigger. Too much stomach acid, a lack of nutrients such as vitamin A (which strengthens the stomach lining), and a high intake of 'irritating' foods such as coffee, alcohol or fried food are some factors which could lead to irritation. One job of stomach acid is to effectively sterilise the stomach, so a lack of it increases the risk of infection with pathogens such as *Helicobacter pylori* (see Chapter 5). Once again, antioxidant nutrients such as beta-carotene, vitamin C and selenium help reduce the risk. Regular garlic consumption is also protective.

PANCREATIC CANCER AND LIVER CANCER

One of the jobs of the pancreas is to produce enzymes to digest foods. This less common type of cancer interferes with digestion, making optimal nutrition difficult. It is often diagnosed after a person starts to experience chronic indigestion and loss of weight. Exactly why it occurs is not known although risk factors do include low intakes of fruit and vegetables, low intake of fibre, high consumption of meat, smoking, and possibly excessive coffee consumption, although not all studies agree.

The liver is the primary organ of detoxification and liver cancer is highly indicative of over-exposure to and/or an inability to detoxify carcinogens. Improving detoxification potential may reduce risk (see Chapter 17). Excess alcohol is the greatest single risk factor, as is use of certain drugs, including Tamoxifen (the most commonly prescribed drug for breast cancer). Certain types of hepatitis also increase the risk.

All the advice in this book for restoring digestive health is ideal for minimising the chance of developing liver cancer, including avoiding coffee and cigarettes, eating plenty of fruit and vegetables and limiting meat and alcohol. In the case of pancreatic cancer, taking digestive enzymes and specially prepared food, soups and juices may be necessary to help digestion and absorption of nutrients.

COLO-RECTAL CANCER

Colo-rectal or bowel cancer is the second most serious cancer in the UK – each year more than 30 000 people are diagnosed with the disease and around 18 000 die of it. If it is detected in its early stages, there is an 85 per cent chance that it can be cured, but unfortunately many people are diagnosed too late. Although between 5 and 10 per cent of sufferers have a genetic predisposition to bowel cancer, there is no doubt that it is linked to diet and lifestyle. Carcinogens in what we eat, exacerbated by putrefying food (because of poor digestion and constipation), and micro-organisms in an unhealthy gut, play a big part. The greatest risk factors are eating a diet high in fat (especially saturated) and meat (especially grilled, barbecued or burnt), and low in fibre, a history of polyps, smoking, excess alcohol, lack of exercise, lack of vegetables, high calorie intake and prolonged stress.

A high-fibre diet shortens the time food takes to pass through the digestive tract and thereby reduces carcinogen exposure. In other words we can minimise our risk of developing colo-rectal cancer by choosing a diet high in fibre, which helps things move along more quickly, and low in meat, which takes longer to digest. Fibre helps to reduce the 'availability' of carcinogenic compounds. Soluble fibre acts as fuel for the growth of friendly bacteria which, in turn, lower the pH (i.e. raise the acidity) of the colon. And higher acidity is associated with a lower risk of developing colo-rectal cancer.

One study examined the faecal pH of South Asian vegetarian pre-menopausal women compared with white vegetarian and white omnivorous women to see whether there was any link between this and their intakes of fibre, fat and cholesterol. The research found that there was indeed an association between high-fibre diets and faecal pH. It also showed that such a diet decreased the concentration of bile acids in faeces, a factor which has been linked to a lowered chance of developing colo-rectal cancer.[16] A high-fat, low-fibre, high refined carbohydrate diet also increases activity of beta-glucoronidase, an enzyme secreted by toxic bacteria, which can generate carcinogens in the colon.[17] The activity of this enzyme can be measured in a stool test such as the Comprehensive Digestive Stool Analysis by Great Smokies Diagnostic Laboratories (see Useful Addresses) which a clinical nutritionist can arrange for you.

The protective effect of cruciferous vegetables (such as Brussels sprouts, cabbage, cauliflower and broccoli) against cancers of the digestive tract is well recognised. A recent double-blind study using Brussels sprouts suggests that the protective mechanism may involve the natural compound glucosinolate. In the study, subjects first ate glucosinolate-containing Brussels sprouts for seven days and then glucosinolate-free sprouts for the same period. After the glucosinolate intake, detoxification enzymes in the colon increased by 30 per cent compared with the glucosinolate-free period.[18] It has been suggested that glucosinolate in cruciferous vegetables enhances the detoxifying enzymes which could increase the body's capacity to withstand the burden of daily exposure to toxins and carcinogens.

Particularly important nutrients are beta-carotene, vitamin C, folic acid, vitamin D, calcium and selenium. Diet, however, is the major prevention factor. Regular garlic consumption reduces the risk, as does live yoghurt because it provides beneficial bacteria to improve intestinal health. Supplementing antioxidant nutrients, such as vitamin C, beta-carotene and vitamin E, has been shown to reverse polyps. Although not all polyps lead on to colo-rectal cancer, certain kinds indicate the beginning of the process which, if not reversed, can eventually result in cancerous growths. So the presence of polyps indicates the need to jump into action with a diet and supplement programme to restore digestive health (see Part 4).

PART 4

RESTORING DIGESTIVE HEALTH

CHAPTER 23

ACTION PLAN FOR HEALTHY DIGESTION

The digestive system is one of the most regenerative parts of the body and in 30 days you can make an incredible difference to your digestive health. Provided you are not suffering from a major digestive problem (in which case I advise you to consult a clinical nutritionist as well as your doctor), the following 30-day programme is a safe, effective and fast way to restore digestive health. It is based on the following four phases:

- **Remove** digestive irritants and allergy-provoking foods
- **Cleanse** the digestive tract
- **Re-inoculate** with beneficial bacteria
- **Rebuild** a healthy digestive tract.

In practical terms, this means following a diet and supplement strategy week by week for four weeks, followed by a digestive health maintenance programme. The first two weeks focus on removing digestive irritants and allergy-provoking foods and cleansing the digestive tract. Supplements include cleansing and detoxifying herbs (explained in Chapter 24). The last two weeks focus on restoring the beneficial bacteria and rebuilding a healthy digestive tract. The diet throughout is The Digestion-Friendly Diet (explained in Chapter 25). Specific details on the digestive supplements, and how and when to take them, are given in Chapter 26.

If you are taking additional nutritional supplements (such as a multivitamin and vitamin C), continue to take these as they support your liver's ability to detoxify. A basic ongoing supplement programme for maintaining digestive health is given in Chapter 26.

The schedule of digestive supplements for each week is shown below. Take these supplements immediately before each meal, together with a large glass of water.

	Breakfast	Lunch	Dinner
Week 1			
Colon-cleansing fibres	2	2	2
Colon-cleansing herbs	1	1	1
Digestive enzymes	–	1	1
Week 2			
Colon-cleansing fibres	2	2	2
Colon-cleansing herbs	1	1	1
Digestive enzymes	–	1	1
Probiotic	–	–	1
Week 3			
Digestive enzymes	–	1	1
Probiotic	1	–	1
L-Glutamine (5g)	–	–	1
Week 4			
Digestive enzymes	–	1	1
Probiotic	1	–	1
L-Glutamine (5g)	–	–	1

CHAPTER 24

Digestive Cleansing

We have all become more and more aware of the increasing pollution in our environment, in our water and food, and the poisons and micro-organisms in our bodies that can lead to disease. Although the human body appears to be a vulnerable and sensitive organism, we have in fact been built to survive in an ocean of toxicity, and we have a number of ways of excluding, detoxifying and eliminating poisons. Only by understanding clearly how we build up toxicity can we reverse the process through cleansing and detoxification.

In 1933, Dr Anthony Bassler wrote, after a 25-year study of over 5000 cases, 'Every physician should realise that the intestinal toxemias are the most important primary and contributing causes of many disorders and diseases of the human body.'[1] Intestinal toxemia, or toxicity, is not a condition that has disappeared. On the contrary, it is very much on the increase.

The process may start by eating poor-quality, even toxic food that contains insufficient nutrients. We digest our food poorly, leaving remains which attract parasitic, pathogenic micro-organisms. Stress and drugs make the situation worse. We develop a putrefactive intestine. The intestinal wall comes under attack and weakens, allowing toxins and half-digested food into the blood. This provokes immune system reactions and exhaustion of the liver. The organs of elimination are overwhelmed, and disease begins from toxicity and low immunity. Reversing this process means countering each of these stages with a method of natural cleansing and healing.

THE DIGESTION-FRIENDLY DIET

The first place to start is your diet. The Western diet has repeatedly been shown to lack vitality and freshness, to be low in fibre and too refined. Industrial food production has led to low levels of vitamins and minerals and high quantities of preservatives and other additives. Meat consumption can raise the putrefactive bacteria and milk can increase the less desirable Streptococcus species of bacteria. Vegetables, on the other hand, promote the beneficial *Lactobacillus acidophilus* and Bifidobacteria. On average, vegetarians and organic food eaters are simply much healthier. The principles of digestion-friendly eating are explained in the next chapter.

DIGESTIVE CLEANSING

Diet alone is neither the quickest nor the most effective way to restore digestive health. In addition to a diet that provides key nutrients and removes digestive irritants, certain herbs and fibres can help to cleanse the digestive tract and calm down inflammation. Combinations of these herbs and fibres are available in a number of 'colon-cleansing' powders and capsules. These are usually taken for two to four weeks and are recommended as part of my programme for restoring digestive health. My favourite remedies are Higher Nature's Colo-Fibre and Colo-Clear (see Useful Addresses), based on the research of Brian Wright, author of the *Colon Health Handbook*.

Colon-cleansing fibres

Not all fibres are the same. Some, such as wheat bran, are quite irritating to the digestive tract and not ideal for restoring digestive health. Special herbal sources of fibre, when mixed with water, act as mucins, or gels, which both add bulk and are soothing because they help to calm down inflammation in the intestines. They also absorb toxic material and help to eliminate it. Brian Wright recommends the following combination of colon-cleansing fibres:

- **Linseed** is a bulking laxative traditionally used to heal intestinal problems. It contains glycosides that prevent muscle spasms, and omega 3 oils which act as natural anti-inflammatory agents.
- **Psyllium husks** are soft, cooling, lubricating, mucus-clearing, diuretic, and absorb poisons.
- **Slippery elm** has a soothing, coating mucilage that protects the intestinal walls from acids and toxins and has been used extensively in the treatment of ulcers and inflammation.
- **Pectin** is a gel from fruit that absorbs toxins, particularly heavy metals and aluminium.
- **Fennel and fenugreek** are also recommended.

This fibre combination can be used indefinitely, or in combination with colon-cleansing herbs. The recommended intake is two Colo-Fibre capsules, three times a day, taken before a meal, together with a large glass of water. This provides around 4g of these fibres.

Colon-cleansing herbs

A number of herbs have been used for generations to help restore digestive health. Modern medicine is starting to identify the active ingredients and actions in these ancient remedies. Brian Wright recommends the following colon-cleansing herbs:

- **Acacia gum** is a protective and anti-inflammatory plant gum.
- **Alfalfa** is used as a traditional intestinal cleanser.
- **Blessed thistle** helps the rebuilding of mucosal wall, and is traditionally used for detoxifying and treating irritable bowel syndrome.
- **Cayenne** has an anti-inflammatory effect.
- **Cloves** are antiseptic, anaesthetic, antispasmodic, anti-inflammatory and reduce intestinal gas.
- **Milk thistle** is a detoxifying herb and a powerful antioxidant, inhibiting inflammation.
- **Red clover** contains anti-inflammatory, antispasmodic glycosides and flavonoids, which are antioxidants and hence help detoxify the body.

This herbal combination, taken over a fortnight or month, in conjunction with colon-cleansing fibres and a digestion-friendly diet, can significantly speed your return to digestive well-being. You need about 2g of a combination of these herbs, which is the equivalent of taking one Colo-Clear capsule three times a day.

COLONIC THERAPY

Another way to speed up digestive cleansing is colonic therapy or colonics. Essentially, this is an extensive enema. Warm water, sometimes containing herbs, is passed very gently and carefully, by a qualified practitioner (see Useful

Addresses), up into the colon from the anus. This softens impacted faecal matter which can then be more easily eliminated. A course of colonic treatments, over a month, can help to speed up detoxification of the body. As most of the contents of the colon are evacuated during this time, including beneficial bacteria, it is important to repopulate the digestive tract with 'friendly' bacteria at the end of the course of colonics by taking probiotic supplements.

One of the great advantages of colonic therapy, administered by a skilled practitioner, is that it can help to re-establish proper peristalsis. Often, as a result of long-term constipation, the proper peristaltic action of muscles surrounding the digestive tract can become suppressed. Exercise, drinking enough water, eating fibre-rich foods and breathing from the belly are also important for maintaining colonic health.

CHAPTER 25

THE DIGESTION-FRIENDLY DIET

Throughout the centuries, health experts have extolled the value of spring-cleaning the body. In much the same way as you need a holiday from work, your body needs a break from detoxifying. One of the traditional methods of purifying the body is fasting. The fact that many people report feeling so much more vital after fasting is testimony to the fact that making energy is as much a result of improving the body's ability to detoxify as it is about eating the right foods.

However, not everybody feels better for fasting and not always right away. A common occurrence is the so-called 'healing crisis' when a person feels worse for a few days and then feels better. What we are learning about detoxification processes suggests that some may be experiencing a health crisis rather than healing crisis. Once the body starts to liberate and eliminate toxic material, if the liver isn't up to the job symptoms of intoxication can result. Hence, modern detox regimes tend to use modified fasts, in which the person is given a low-toxin diet, plus plenty of the key nutrients needed to speed up the body's ability to detoxify.

Doing this once a year, for a couple of weeks, can make a

major difference to your energy levels. A more focused approach would involve consulting a clinical nutritionist (see Useful Addresses) and having a comprehensive detoxification profile test. On the basis of this, they will devise a specific diet and supplement programme designed to restore optimal detoxification potential. I have seen many long-term sufferers of chronic fatigue syndrome completely recover within weeks of implementing a nutritional programme specifically designed to improve their detoxification potential. I am convinced that the vast majority of people with chronic fatigue syndrome can be helped in this way.

DETOXIFICATION

Obviously, the first step to detoxifying the body is to remove or lessen the toxic load. Some foods are almost entirely toxin-generating, while others are very detoxifying. Most, however, have good factors and bad factors.

The best detoxifying foods

Fruit More or less all fruits are good for detoxification, but the most beneficial fruits with the highest detox potential include: fresh apricots, all types of berries, cantaloupe, citrus fruits, kiwi, papaya, peaches, mango, melons and red grapes. Go easy on bananas, one a day only. Dried fruit is best avoided during these two weeks.

Vegetables All are great, but the following are especially good: artichokes, peppers, beetroot, Brussels sprouts, broccoli, red cabbage, carrots, cauliflower, cucumber, kale, pumpkin, spinach, sweet potato, tomato, watercress. White potatoes and avocado should be eaten in moderation.

Also excellent are sprouted beans and seeds. Try alfalfa, sprouted mung beans, chickpeas, lentils, aduki beans and sprouted sunflower seeds. These are available to buy ready-sprouted in most healthfood shops and some supermarkets and greengrocers.

These foods should make up the bulk of your two-week detox diet. Needless to say, choose organic wherever possible so your body doesn't have to detoxify the pesticides.

Supplementary detoxifying foods

The following foods are generally good for you, but may contain low levels of toxins. These should make up no more than a third of your two-week diet.

Grains Choose brown rice, corn, millet, quinoa.

Fish Salmon, mackerel, sardines and tuna.

Meat Organic skinless chicken, turkey and wild game.

Oils Use extra-virgin olive oil for cooking and in place of butter, and cold-pressed seed oils for dressing. Organic, cold-pressed flax oil is the best for this.

Nuts and Seeds Have a large handful a day of raw, unsalted nuts and seeds. Try grinding them up and sprinkling them over fruit salad. Include almonds, Brazils, hazelnuts, pecans, pumpkin seeds, sunflower seeds, sesame seeds and flax seeds.

Foods to avoid while detoxifying

The following foods, while normally OK in moderation, are best avoided during the two weeks because they are hard to digest, mildly irritate the gut or are hard to detoxify.

Gluten grains Barley, oats, rye and wheat (including wheat bran, spelt and kamut).

Meat and dairy produce Milk and all dairy products, eggs and organic red meat.

Harmful foods

The following foods should be avoided at all times:

- red meat
- refined foods (e.g. white bread/pasta/rice)
- sugar and any foods containing it
- salt and any foods containing it
- hydrogenated or partially hydrogenated fat
- artificial sweeteners
- food additives and preservatives (a good general rule – if you can't pronounce it, avoid it!)
- alcohol
- tea and coffee
- all fizzy drinks, including cola drinks and squash

As far as you can, also avoid: chilli, fried foods, pesticides, exhaust fumes and medications (most contain harmful substances that require detoxification).

Detox drinks

Needless to say, during these two weeks alcohol is out. It is a major toxin for the body. So too are any sources of 'methyl-xanthines', a family of chemicals that includes caffeine, tannin, theobromine and theophylline. This means no chocolate, coffee, tea and no peppermint tea either. Alternatives are shown below.

- Fruit juice – ideally freshly made, and always diluted with an equal quantity of water.
- Aqua Libra, Amé and elderflower champagne for special occasions!
- Herbal teas – there is now a huge variety to choose from; sample a few until you find the one you like best.
- Rooibosch tea – caffeine-free and tastes very similar to 'normal' tea.
- Dandelion coffee can be drunk as a coffee replacement whilst you are on your two-week detox diet. Once it is complete, try Caro, Barleycup and Teechino.

The best drink of all is pure water and lots of it. Drink 2 litres of purified, distilled, filtered or bottled water a day. This may seem like an awful lot. However, water puts no burden on the body and helps to dilute toxins as they are eliminated.

DIGESTION-FRIENDLY RECIPES

Below is a selection of delicious meal ideas taken from my *Optimum Nutrition Cookbook,* co-written with Judy Ridgway (see Recommended Reading). The recipes are based on fresh, healthy ingredients that are naturally rich in nutrients that aid digestion, and they are largely free from digestive irritants. This will give you plenty of ideas for putting the digestion-friendly diet into practice.

BREAKFASTS

Berry Booster
Rice Flake Porridge
Healthy Scrambled Eggs
Quinoa Porridge with Bananas
The Ultimate Power Breakfast
Mixed Cereal Muesli with Grated Apples or Pears

LIGHT MEALS

Winter Salad Platter with Tangy Cucumber Dressing
Lemon Chicken on Leafy Asparagus Salad
Steam-fry Vegetables with Green Curry Paste
Spanish Rice with Fennel
Warm Mackerel Salad with Avocado and Mango and Honey-Toasted Sunflower Seeds
Devilled Tomatoes on Polenta Squares
Hot Sour Prawn Soup

MAIN COURSES

Vegetarian Kebabs with Barbecue Sauce and Brown Rice
Garden Paella
Red Mullet Baked in a Paper Case
Vegetable Parcels with Kiwi Salsa
Flash-Grilled Tuna in a Lemon Ginger Marinade with Quinoa and Red Pepper Salsa
Indian Vegan Feast
Duck Slivers with Orange Beansprouts

DESSERTS

Sweet Potato and Ginger Soufflé
Baked Apples with Seville Orange Marmalade
Papaya Cups with Strawberries and Lime
Raisin and Vanilla Tofucake
Date and Orange Flan
Fruit Crumble

DRINKS

Lemon Ginger Punch
Watermelon Whizz
Berry Juice Cocktail
Mango and Banana Dream
Omega Drink

CHAPTER 26

DIGESTIVE SUPPLEMENTS

Nutritional supplements, taken on a regular basis, make a big difference to your digestive health. This is because every step of the digestive process, from digestion to detoxification, depends on a whole host of nutrients that are often deficient in our modern diet.

To help you find your way through the maze of natural digestive remedies, here is a summary of the key supplements you are likely to encounter, or be recommended if you consult a clinical nutritionist. Depending on your health problem, these supplements may be worth taking as part of your strategy for restoring digestive health.

For recommended 'Basic' and 'Digestive Healing' dosage levels, see pages 168–9.

VITAMIN AND MINERAL SUPPLEMENTS

The basis of any supplement programme is a good high-strength multivitamin and mineral. This will contain basic levels of vitamins A, B, C, D and E plus minerals such as calcium, magnesium, iron, zinc, manganese, chromium and selenium. These nutrients support digestion, thus maintaining a healthy digestive tract and liver detoxification. Multivitamins never provide enough vitamin C so I also recommend supplementing 1000mg of vitamin C. Also helpful are additional antioxidant nutrients. These protect against oxidant damage to the digestive tract and are vital in detoxifying the body. In addition to vitamins A, C and E and the antioxidant minerals zinc and selenium, good antioxidants should also provide a source of glutathione or cysteine and flavonoids such as berry extracts.

PROBIOTICS

It is not necessary to take probiotic supplements every day: they are the best way to re-inoculate the digestive tract with beneficial bacteria after an infection or as part of a strategy for restoring digestive health. There are many different strains of health-promoting bacteria (see Chapter 13) but the two main ones are *Lactobacillus acidophilus* and Bifidobacteria. Make sure these are present in reasonable quantities, such as 100 million or more viable organisms per capsule or serving. Better supplements also contain fructo-oligosaccharides (FOS) which help the bacteria to multiply once they are inside you. Special strains of bacteria are most beneficial for children. These include *B. infantis*. Good for both adults and children is *Lactobacillus salivarius*, which attaches to the intestinal wall and has been shown to reduce the number of pathogenic organisms.[2]

DIGESTIVE ENZYMES

These include a wide variety of enzymes from both animal and plant sources. What you are after is a supplement that contains lipase (for digesting fat), protease (for digesting protein), amylase (for digesting carbohydrate), cellulase (for digesting cellulose), amyloglucosidase (for digesting glucosides in certain vegetables), and possibly lactase (for digesting milk sugar). You need around 20mg of each to make a difference to your digestion. Papain, from papaya, digests protein; as does bromelain from pineapple. These are alternative sources of protease enzymes. If you are lacking stomach acid you can supplement betaine hydrochloride, at around 300mg a day, with meals. To further help fat digestion, supplement lecithin, either as granules or capsules.

SUPPLEMENTS FOR SPECIFIC DIGESTIVE PURPOSES

Intestinal repair and rebuilding

A number of supplements exist to help intestinal rebuilding and repair. The key nutrients are vitamin A and zinc. Certain forms of zinc can be irritating to the digestive tract in large amounts. I recommend zinc citrate, ascorbate or amino acid chelate. Glutamine is direct fuel for the intestinal mucosa and a great gut healer. You need 5–10g a day, best taken last thing at night. Supplements are very expensive, but you can buy this amino acid as a powder. Butyric acid, a non-essential fat normally made by intestinal bacteria, also acts as fuel for the intestinal mucosa. You need around 500mg or more a day. Essential fats, especially the omega 3 fats, help reduce inflammation.

Antispasmodic

Peppermint oil capsules are available as an antispasmodic, which means they help calm down muscular contraction in the digestive tract.

Constipation

For the immediate relief of constipation, herbal remedies containing either senna or cascara are available. These are mild irritants and are best used only in the short term. A less drastic way to solve such a problem is to supplement fructo-oligosaccharides (FOS) which increase the transit time by maintaining a higher moisture level in the digestive tract. You need about 5g a day.

Infection fighters

There are many remedies specifically designed to give unfavourable micro-organisms a hard time. These vary depending on the infection and may include caprylic acid, grapefruit seed extract, artemesia, goldenseal, olive leaf extract, garlic and many others (see Chapter 14). Consult a nutritionist or herbalist to determine the best dosage levels for your particular digestive problem.

Detox supplements

Some supplements focus specifically on improving the body's ability to detoxify (see Chapter 17). The nutrients needed to support Phase 1 of detoxification are vitamins B2, B3, B6, B12, folic acid, glutathione, branched chain amino acids, flavonoids and phospholipids, plus a good supply of antioxidant nutrients to disarm dangerous intermediary oxidants created during this stage. Phase 2 of detoxification can be triggered by a specific list of nutrients, including the amino acids glycine, taurine, glutamine and arginine. Cysteine, N-acetyl cysteine and methionine are also precursors for these nutrients (i.e. the body can convert these into the others). Combinations of these nutrients are available, together with detoxifying herbs such as milk thistle (which contains Silymarin).

The following levels of key nutrients serve as a guide to what you need for optimal digestive health. The 'Basic' levels apply to everybody. The levels recommended 'For Digestive Healing' are a rough guide only. What you need depends on your particular problem. Either see the relevant chapter in this book for specific guidance or follow the Action Plan for Healthy Digestion (see pages 150–1).

Nutrient	Basic	For Digestive Healing
Vitamins		
Vitamin A	15 000ius	20 000–35 000ius
as retinol	7500ius	7500–15 000ius
as beta-carotene	7500ius	12 500–20 000ius
Vitamin C	1000mg	2000–4000mg
Vitamin D	400ius	
Vitamin E	150mg (200iu)	400mg (500iu)
B1 (Thiamine)	25mg	
B2 (Riboflavin)	25mg	
B3 (Niacin)	25mg	50mg
B5 (Pantothenic acid)	25mg	
B6 (Pyridoxine)	25mg	50mg
B12	10mcg	
Folic acid	100mcg	
Biotin	50mcg	
Minerals		
Calcium	350mg	500mg
Magnesium	200mg	500mg
Zinc	15mg	25mg
Iron	10mg	
Manganese	5mg	
Chromium	50mcg	
Selenium	100mcg	200mcg
Amino Acids		
Reduced glutathione	50mg	100mg
or N-Acetyl-Cysteine	500mg	1000mg
Glutamine		5000–10 000mg

Nutrient	Basic	For Digestive Healing
Fats		
EPA		360–3000mg (1000mg)
GLA		250mg
Butyric acid		500mg
Enzymes		
Protease		20mg
Amylase		20mg
Lipase		20mg
Amyloglucosidase		10mg
Betaine hydrochloride		300mg
Papain		100mg
Bromelain		100mg
Beneficial Bacteria		
Lactobacillus acidophilus		100–500 million organisms
Bifidobacteria		100–500 million organisms
Other		
Co-enzyme Q10		30mg
Lecithin		2400mg

In practical terms the easiest way to achieve the basic levels of these nutrients is to take:

- a good, all-round multivitamin and mineral
- 1000mg of vitamin C
- an antioxidant complex containing glutathione or N-acetyl-cysteine
- plus 'extras' such as digestive enzymes, probiotics, glutamine or detox formulas.

References

Part 1

1 CNEAT (Council for Nutrition Education and Therapy) Survey 1990.

2 Rafsky, H.A. and Weingarten, M., 'The study of the gastric secretory response in the aged', *Gastroenterology*, May, pp 348–52 (1947).
Baker, H. et al., 'Oral versus intramuscular vitamin supplementation for hypovitaminosis in the elderly', *J Am Geriat Soc*, vol 48, pp 42–5 (1980).

3 Slomianye, A. et al., *Gut*, vol 35 (71), (1994).
Niederhauser, A. et al., *Gut*, vol 35 (1427), (1994).

4 Leoci, E. and Lerardi, E., *Gut*, vol 35 (78), (1994).

Part 2

1 Pfeiffer, C., original research paper (unpublished), Brain BioCenter.
Pillay, D. et al., 'Zinc status in vitamin B6 deficiency', *Int J Vitam Nutr Res*, vol 67 (1), pp 22–6 (1997).

2 Mitsuuoka, T., 'Intestinal flora & aging', *Nutr Rev*, vol 50 (12), pp 438–46 (1992).

3 Bernet, M.F. et al., '*Lactobacillus acidophilus* LA1 binds to cultured human intestinal cell lines and inhibits cell attachment and cell invasion by enterovirulent bacteria', *Gut*, vol 35, pp 483–9 (1994).

4 Peltonen, R. et al., 'Changes of faecal flora in rheumatoid arthritis during fasting and one-year vegetarian diet', *Br J Rheumatol*, vol 33, pp 638–43 (1994).

5 Majamaa, H. and Isolaui, E., 'Probiotics: a novel approach in the management of food allergy', *J Allergy Clin Immunol*, vol 99, pp 179–85 (1997).
6 Hunter, J.O., 'Food allergy – or enterometabolic disorder?' *Lancet*, vol 338, pp 495–6 (1991).
7 Goel, R.K. et al., 'Anti-ulcerogenic effect of banana powder (Musa sapientum var. paradisiaca) and its effect on mucosal resistance', *J Ethnopharmacol*, vol 18 (1), pp 33–44 (1986).
8 *Am J Clin Nutr*, vol 65 (1997).
9 *New Scientist*, 17 Dec 1994.
10 Bjarnason et al., *Lancet*, vol 1, p 297 (1983).
11 Ryan, A.J. et al., 'Gastrointestinal permeability following aspirin intake and prolonged running', *Med Sci Sports Exercise*, vol 28 (6), pp 698–705 (1996).
12 Allison et al., *N Engl J Med*, vol 327, pp 749–54 (1992).
13 Kulkarni, R.R. et al., 'Treatment of osteo-arthritis with a herbo-mineral formulation: a double blind, placebo controlled, cross over study', *J Ethnopharmacol*, vol 33 (1–2), pp 91–5 (1991).
14 Joe, B. et al., 'Presence of an acidic glycoprotein in the serum of arthritic rats: modulation by capsaicin and curcumin', *Mol Cell Biochem*, vol 169 (1–2), pp 125–34 (1997).
15 McCarthy, G.M. and Mc Carty, D.J., 'Effect of topical capsaicin in the therapy of painful osteoarthritis of the hands', *J Rheumatol*, vol 19, pp 604–7 (1992).
16 Curcuminoids – the active principles from turmeric root', Sabinsa Corporation.
17 Catassi et al., *Acta Paediatr*, vol 84, pp 672–6 (1995).
18 ION research by Leonie Buswell (1996).
19 *J Am Ger Soc*, vol 45 (1997).
20 US News and World Report 20 Feb 1989, vol 106 (7), 77 (2).

Part 3

1 Drossman, D.A. et al., 'US house-holder survey of functional GI disorders: prevalence, sociodemography and health impact', *Dig Dis Sci*, vol 38, pp 1569–80 (1993).
2 Thorne, G.M., *Infect Dis Clin North Am*, vol 2 (3), pp 747–51 (1988).

3 Wolfe, M.S., *Clin Microbiology Review*, vol 5 (1), pp 93–100 (1992).

4 Eastham, E.J. et al., 'Diagnosis of *Giardia lamblia* infection as a cause of diarrhoea', *Lancet*, pp 950–51 (1976).

5 Bueno, Hermann, *Uninvited Guests*, Keats (1996).

6 Wynburn-Mason, R., *The Causation of Rheumatoid Disease and Many Human Cancers: A New Concept in Medicine*, Iji Publishing Company, Tokyo (1978).

7 Russo, A.R. et al., 'Presumptive evidence for *Blastocystis hominis* as a cause of colitis', *Arch Intern Med*, vol 148 (5), p 1064 (1988).
Hussain Quadri, S.M., Al-Okaili, G.A. and Al-Dayel, F., 'Clinical significance of *Blastocystis hominis*, *J Clin Microbiol*, vol 27 (11), pp 2407–9 (1989).
Kain, K.C. et al., 'Epidemiology and clinical features associated with *Blastocystis hominis* infection', *Diagn Microbiol Infect Dis*, vol 8 (4), pp 234–44 (1987).

8 Galland, L., 'Leaky Gut Syndrome: Breaking the vicious cycle', *Townsend Letter for Doctors* (Aug/Sept 1995).

9 Northrop-Clewes, C.A. and Downes, R.M., 'Chronic diarrhoea and malnutrition in the Gambia: studies on intestinal permeability', *Trans R Soc Trop Med Hyg*, vol 85 (1), pp 8–11 (1991).

10 Sudduth, W.H., 'The role of bacteria and enterotoxemia in physical addition to alcohol', *Microecology and Therapy*, vol 18 (1989).

11 Bernard, et al., 'Increased intestinal permeability in bronchial asthma', *Allergy Clin Immunol*, vol 97, pp 1173–8 (1996).

12 Andre, C. et al., *Ann Allergy*, vol 59 (11), pp 127–30 (1987).
Andre, C. et al., *Ann Allergy*, vol 44 (9), pp 47–51 (1989).

13 Pearson, A. et al., 'Intestinal permeability in children with Crohn's disease and coeliac disease', *BMJ*, vol 285, p 20 (1982).

14 Sanderson, I.R. et al., 'Improvement of abnormal lactulose/rhamnose permeability in active Crohn's disease of the small bowel by an elemental diet', *Gut*, vol 28, pp 1073–6 (1987).

15 Jacobs, E.J. and White, E., 'Constipation, laxative use and colon cancer among middle-aged adults', *Epidemiology*, vol 9 (4), pp 385–91 (1998).

16 Reddy, S. et al., 'Faecal pH, bile acid and sterol concentrations in premenopausal Indian and white vegetarian compared with white omnivores', *Br J Nutr*, vol 79, pp 495–500 (1998).

17 Hambly, R.J. et al., 'Effects of high- and low-risk diets on gut microflora-associated biomarkers of colon cancer in human flora-associated rats', *Nutr Cancer*, vol 27 (3), pp 250–5 (1997).
18 *Carcinogenesis*, vol 16 (1995).

Part 4

1 Bassler, A., 'Intestinal toxemia', *Medical Journal and Record*, vol 136 (1933).
2 Cole, C.B. and Fuller, R., 'A note . . . on the coliform population of the neonatal rat gut', *J Appl Bacteriology*, vol 56 (3), (1984).

RECOMMENDED READING

Baker MD, Sidney MacDonald, *Detoxification and Healing*, Keats Publishing, 1997

Bland PhD, Jeffrey, *The 20-Day Rejuvenation Diet Programme*, Keats Publishing, 1997

Crook, Dr William, *The Yeast Connection*, Vintage Books, 1986

Galland, Dr Leo, *Power Healing*, Random House, 1998

Holford, Patrick, *The Optimum Nutrition Bible*, Piatkus, 1997

Holford, Patrick, *100% Health*, Piatkus, 1998

Holford, Patrick and Ridgway, Judy, *The Optimum Nutrition Cookbook*, Piatkus, 1999

White, Erica, *The Beat Candida Cookbook*, Thorsons, 1999

Useful Addresses

Diagnostic Laboratories
I recommend that you visit a clinical nutritionist who can arrange for you to have any of a number of biochemical tests done. Collection kits (containing swabs, specimen bottles and even small proctoscopes for taking rectal swabs, plus full instructions for doctor and patient) are available free of charge from these labs. Both Parascope and Great Smokies will provide you with a photograph of any parasites identified in the stool sample.

Parascope Laboratory
Tel: 0113 392 4657.

Diagnos-Techs
Tel: 01792 464911.

Great Smokies Diagnostic Laboratory
Agents in the UK are Health Interlink. *Tel:* 01582 794 094.

Biolab
Tel: 020 7636 5959.

Digestive Disorders Foundation
3 St Andrews Place, London NW1 4LB. *Tel:* 020 7486 0341

Psychocalisthenics is an excellent exercise system that takes less than twenty minutes a day, and develops strength, suppleness and stamina and generates vital energy. The best way to learn it is to do the Psychocalisthenics Training. See www.patrickholford.com (seminars) for details on this or call 020 8871 2949. Also available is the book *Master Level Exercise, Psychocalisthenics*, and the Psychocalisthenics CD and DVD. For further information please see www.pcals.com.

Biocare produce a wide range of supplements, including DigestPro. *Tel:* 0121 433 3727 or visit www.biocare.co.uk.

Solgar produce a wide range of products available through health-food shops. For your nearest stockist, contact Solgar Vitamins Ltd, Aldbury, Tring, Herts HP23 5PT. *Tel:* 01442 890355.

Nutrition Consultations

For a personal referral by Patrick Holford to a nutritional therapist in your area, visit www.patrickholford.com and select 'consultations' for an immediate online referral. This service gives details on whom to see in the UK as well as internationally. If there is no-one available nearby you can always do an online assessment – see below.

Nutrition Assessment Online

You can have your own personal health and nutrition assessment online using the 100% Health Programme. Visit www.patrickholford.com and to go 'consultations'.

Institute for Optimum Nutrition (ION)

ION offers a three-year foundation degree course in nutritional therapy that includes training in the optimum nutrition approach to mental health. There is a clinic, a list of nutrition practitioners across the UK, an information service and a quarterly journal – Optimum Nutrition. Contact ION at Avalon House, 72 Lower Mortlake Road, Richmond TW9 2JY, or visit www.ion.ac.uk. *Tel:* 020 8877 9993.

INDEX